Understanding
Skin Problems

Understanding Illness and Health

Many health problems and worries are strongly influenced by our thoughts and feelings. These exciting new books, written by experts in the psychology of health, are essential reading for sufferers, their families and friends.

Each book presents objective, easily understood information and advice about what the problem is, the treatments available and, most importantly, how your state of mind can help or hinder the way you cope. You will discover how to have a positive, hopeful outlook, which will help you choose the most effective treatment for you and your particular lifestyle, with confidence.

The series is edited by JANE OGDEN, Reader in Health Psychology, Guy's, King's and St Thomas' School of Medicine, King's College London, UK

Titles in the series

KAREN BALLARD   Understanding Menopause

SIMON DARNLEY & BARBARA MILLAR   Understanding Irritable Bowel Syndrome

LINDA PAPADOPOULOS & CARL WALKER   Understanding Skin Problems

PENNY TITMAN   Understanding Childhood Eczema

Understanding Skin Problems

Acne, Eczema, Psoriasis and
Related Conditions

LINDA PAPADOPOULOS AND CARL WALKER
London Metropolitan University, UK

WILEY

Copyright © 2003   John Wiley & Sons Ltd, The Atrium, Southern Gate, Chichester, West Sussex PO19 8SQ, England

Telephone (+44) 1243 779777

Email (for orders and customer service enquiries): cs-books@wiley.co.uk
Visit our Home Page on www.wileyeurope.com or www.wiley.com

Reprinted August 2003

Other Wiley Editorial Offices

John Wiley & Sons Inc., 111 River Street, Hoboken, NJ 07030, USA

Jossey-Bass, 989 Market Street, San Francisco, CA 94103-1741, USA

Wiley-VCH Verlag GmbH, Boschstr. 12, D-69469 Weinheim, Germany

John Wiley & Sons Australia Ltd, 33 Park Road, Milton, Queensland 4064, Australia

John Wiley & Sons (Asia) Pte Ltd, 2 Clementi Loop #02-01, Jin Xing Distripark, Singapore 129809

John Wiley & Sons Canada Ltd, 22 Worcester Road, Etobicoke, Ontario, Canada M9W 1L1

Wiley also publishes its books in a variety of electronic formats. Some content that appears in print may not be available in electronic books.

Library of Congress Cataloging-in-Publication Data

Papadopoulos, Linda.
  Understanding skin problems : acne, eczema, psoriasis, and related conditions / Linda Papadopoulos and Carl Walker.
     p. ; cm. – (Understanding illness & health)
Includes bibliographical references and index.
  ISBN 0-470-84518-X (pbk. : alk. paper)
 1. Skin – Diseases – Psychological aspects.
  [DNLM: 1. Skin Diseases – psychology – Popular Works. WR 140 P213u 2003] I. Walker, Carl. II. Title. III. Series.
  RL72 .P26 2003
  616.5'01'9 – dc21
                                        2002153122

British Library Cataloguing in Publication Data

A catalogue record for this book is available from the British Library

ISBN 0-470-84518-X

Typeset in 9.5/13pt Photina by Laserwords Private Limited, Chennai, India
Printed and bound in Great Britain by TJ International, Padstow, Cornwall
This book is printed on acid-free paper responsibly manufactured from sustainable forestry in which at least two trees are planted for each one used for paper production.

Contents

About the authors

DR LINDA PAPADOPOULOS is a Reader in Psychology at London Metropolitan University with specific research interests in the field of psychodermatology, and she has consistently published in this field. Dr Papadopoulos is a chartered health and counselling psychologist who has worked in primary care settings as well as maintaining her research group. She also has extensive media commitments, appearing regularly on television and writing her monthly column in *Cosmopolitan* magazine.

CARL WALKER is a Research Psychologist at London Metropolitan University where he is currently finishing a PhD in psychodermatology. He graduated in biology from Royal Holloway and Bedford New College, University of London. His research focuses on body image and disfigurement and the use of psychological therapy in medical contexts. Within this field, he has a particular interest in the psychological aspects of child skin disease and the family.

Introduction

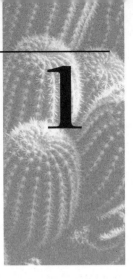

It is estimated that approximately 20 per cent of the UK population suffers with some form of skin disease at any given time, with eczema, acne and infectious disorders (e.g. athlete's foot) being the most commonly presenting complaints to general practitioners (GPs) and dermatologists.

Approximately 15–20 per cent of a GP's workload and 6 per cent of hospital outpatient referrals are for skin problems. Skin disease is also the most frequent reason for sick leave from work and is the most common industrial disease (Gawkrodger, 1997). Yet, in a society where there is so much emphasis placed on looks and appearance, there seems to be little attention given to the psychological effects of skin conditions and the challenges faced by those who suffer from them. From dealing with staring and rude comments to thinking about how to ask the doctor for a referral, people may experience different challenges when living with their skin condition. Unfortunately however, since skin diseases are rarely life-threatening, their impact is often minimised both by family members and by health professionals. As a consequence, a person may feel that they aren't allowed to be upset or even to take time out to cope with their condition. We hope that this book will enable people to address their concerns in a constructive and helpful way. This book addresses principles that are pertinent to all skin diseases, but focuses specifically on acne, eczema, psoriasis and vitiligo, drawing on patients' accounts of living with and coping with their skin disease.

How is skin disease different from other conditions?

Over our years of experience in counselling patients in medical settings it has always struck us how illnesses (and consequently their impact) are assessed in terms of their severity. The assumption is made that the more severe a condition is, the more severe the psychological impact will be on the patient. As a consequence, skin diseases that are rarely life-threatening or physically handicapping, are thought not to pose much of a problem for those that experience them. The fact of the matter is that the severity of a condition is not directly related to how we cope

1

psychologically. Rather, a multitude of factors, including individual coping style, social support, illness beliefs, social stigma and past experience with the illness, all impact on how well we cope.

As with any illness, a skin disease brings on a variety of life changes and challenges that we may not be prepared to deal with. However, unlike conditions which do not change the way people look, skin problems raise a whole new set of challenges because of their visibility. The visibility of certain conditions may attract attention in social situations, thus making the individual feel that they can't keep their condition private or personal. Furthermore, owing to a lack of health education and awareness in dermatology, some people associate skin disease with contagion or lack of hygiene. This ignorance regarding skin conditions means that a skin disease patient may find that some people react negatively towards them or treat them differently because of the way that they look. In many cases the physical changes that may result from skin disease can have a negative effect on body image. Body image is our perception of the way that others see us, and therefore any sudden changes to the way that we look will have an affect on our body image.

As skin diseases are not that well known or understood by the general public, it is quite likely that people's beliefs about various dermatological conditions and the way that people cope with them might be wrong.

Counselling

So far, we have briefly looked at how people can be affected by their skin condition, we now consider how counselling can address and respond to some of these issues. In recent years, health care professionals have recognised that people with medical conditions and their families can be helped, through psychological counselling, to cope more effectively with their illness. Counselling in health care settings for people with medical conditions can specifically:

(1) Help you understand your illness better.

(2) Address your concerns.

(3) Address the family's concerns.

(4) Give the you and your family useful coping strategies.

(5) Help improve compliance with treatment.

(6) Reduce psychological problems associated with your condition.

(7) Help you to communicate better with other health care professionals.

Counselling can also help people make sense of their condition; since many skin conditions have an uncertain cause, people often construct personal accounts to 'explain' their condition. Some of these explanations may have a negative effect on adjustment, depending on the nature of an individual's beliefs. Part of helping people cope with their condition is therefore about making sure that mistaken beliefs about the cause of the illness or guilt don't get in the way of helping them cope. Counselling can also help to normalise people's feelings. Dermatology patients may be referred for counselling because they are finding it difficult to cope with their condition. Feelings of sadness or guilt about not being able to deal with something that others may view as trivial may prompt a referral for counselling, which in turn can help to provide both practical methods for coping with the effects of skin disease and a safe environment where patients can explore their feelings.

About the book

In this book we set out to address some of the core issues that people living with skin disease face. In Chapter 2 we begin with an examination of the commonly held myths about skin disease and the way in which these myths and portrayals of beauty in the media can make skin disease patients feel stigmatised. It is surprising how many of our strongly held beliefs about certain conditions have their basis in superstition and folklore. We unravel myth from fact and we discuss the origins of many of today's views on skin disease.

In Chapter 3 we turn our attention to the actual medical facts concerning skin disease, investigating the causes, prevalence and treatment of different conditions. Chapter 4 is dedicated to examining the concept of coping and the psychological adaptation to skin conditions. In particular we explore ways to cope with difficult social interactions. In Chapter 5 we look at how skin diseases affect relationships and ways that we can improve our interactions with others.

In Chapter 6 we examine the psychological effects of skin disease on children and young people and describe ways for carers and young people themselves to cope with their condition. In Chapter 7 we focus specifically on skin disease patients' relationship with health professionals, giving advice about the best ways to get answers to their questions and where to find the best health professional. In Chapter 8 we take a look at some of the most successful coping strategies that psychologists use to help people cope with skin disease. We take a step-by-step approach to the theory and practical aspects behind each model and discuss useful techniques for finding suitable therapists.

Chapter 9 we call our 'How do I ... ?' chapter where we answer some of the most commonly asked questions from patients and their families, from issues concerning coping in specific situations to addressing the use of herbal remedies. A list of the various associations and help groups that exist around the UK, and a summary of the different services they offer, is given in the 'Useful addresses' section at the back of the book.

The main focus of this book is to describe:

- The psychological impact of dermatological conditions.
- The effects of skin disease on social and familial relationships.
- How to recognise psychological problems associated with skin disease.
- The use of psychological counselling with dermatology patients.

Our hope is that this book will provide you with ideas about how to understand and cope with your condition and also make you better equipped to deal with social situations. We want to end this chapter on a positive note by saying that many people living with illnesses get on with their lives and live happy and fulfilled lives irrespective of their skin condition. It is important to acknowledge, however, that everyone reacts differently to challenges in life and this book may be useful for those who find certain aspects of living with their own or a family member's skin condition challenging. You may wish to use the book as a source of information or just for general interest, but it is important that we convey an understanding of the ways in which dermatology patients can be affected by their condition and the importance of the mind–body connection in the treatment of skin disease.

Summary

- For those that have lived with the consequences of skin disease it is obvious that the effects are more than skin deep.

- There are both social and psychological consequences of living with a skin disease.

- Counselling can play a role in helping people to cope with skin disease.

Myths about skin disease, the media and stigma

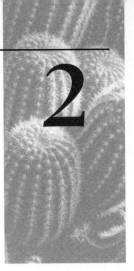

This chapter will outline the common myths about skin disease and the ways in which the media can affect these. We will then look at the ways in which people can feel stigmatised as a result of these myths.

Unlike conditions such as cancer and HIV, which are ranked high on the list of medical problems in terms of public awareness, dermatological conditions rarely receive attention in public health campaigns and so their effect on people's lives tends to be underrated. Furthermore, this lack of awareness means that less is known about the causes and consequences of skin diseases as compared to other, more high profile, medical conditions. It is estimated that approximately 20 per cent of the UK population suffer with some form of skin disease at any time, with eczema, acne and infectious disorders (e.g. athlete's foot) being the most commonly presented complaints at GP's surgeries.

What do people believe about skin diseases: common myths

Skin disease, as is the case with most other medical conditions that alter physical appearance, was viewed in the past as a form of punishment. People have also explained it in terms of a 'wrongdoing' of either the sufferer or their family. This view that some form of magical external force may be responsible for punishing 'bad' people with some kind of deformity dates back thousands of years. The stigmatising nature of conditions such as leprosy, for example, have their roots in the belief that sufferers are unclean, contagious or unable to care for themselves. People with skin diseases have historically been treated as second-class citizens, avoided, pitied and shunned.

These negative reactions to people who have suffered with some form of skin condition were born out of the belief that they were in some way responsible for their misfortune. Stigmatisation is associated with many forms of disfigurement and is sometimes underscored by popular images portrayed in magazines and on television. From fairy tales to soap operas, villains are generally depicted as having not only deviant personalities but also 'deviant' physical characteristics. Heroes, however, seem to be portrayed as flawless and beautiful.

Although mistaken ideas about the causes of skin conditions are now less common, misconceptions and myths still abound about many of them. These are often related to the type of skin condition. For instance, acne is sometimes associated with immaturity or a lack of cleanliness and reactions to this can range from pity to disgust. Reactions about skin condition tend to develop out of beliefs about:

- How the person developed the condition.
- The course of the condition (i.e. will it come and go or will it be permanent?).
- Whether it is treatable.
- Common views and stereotypes about the condition.
- Its location, colour, size or shape.
- The relationship to the affected person.

Listed in Box 1 are some very common misconceptions about skin disease in general. The existence of these mistaken beliefs can seriously affect the way some sufferers of skin conditions think and feel about themselves, more of which will be discussed later.

Box 1. **Common misconceptions about skin disease.**

- Because most skin conditions are not life-threatening, they do not pose a big problem for the patient.
- If the condition is not physically handicapping, then the person's activities and daily routine can't be affected.
- The consequences that a skin disease has on the sufferer's life must be directly related to how severe the condition is.
- Everyone with a skin condition is affected in the same way, regardless of sex, age or race.
- There is no difference in how people react to different skin conditions.

In the following sections some of the common misconceptions about specific skin diseases are outlined.

Myths about acne

- **Acne is related to diet** – no evidence exists to suggest that any particular foods directly cause acne.
- **Acne results from a person's inability to 'properly take care of themselves'** – acne is actually due to inherited factors that increase the production of a substance called sebum and has nothing to do with how a person 'takes care of themselves'.
- **Strong cleansers and constant scrubbing are helpful** – this can actually lead to increased inflammation; mild non-abrasive cleansing is best.
- **Acne is just a stage that people go through during adolescence** – acne may actually begin in or continue through adult life and can affect a person's self-esteem whatever the age of onset.

Myths about eczema

- **Frequent bathing of the affected areas is helpful and soothing** – frequent bathing and long, hot showers should be avoided; moisturising preparations instead of soaps should be used and moisturisers also applied liberally after bathing should be helpful.
- **Eczema is contagious** – eczema is not contagious, and one can't acquire the condition by coming into contact with eczema sufferers or their belongings.
- **Only children get eczema** – although it is common in children, the condition is often seen later in life.

Myths about vitiligo

- **Vitiligo is closely related to leprosy** – vitiligo has long been associated with leprosy due to the fact that leprosy may also appear as white patches that can look like vitiligo. However, the two are *not* connected in any way. Leprosy is contagious whereas vitiligo is genetically determined and not contagious.
- **Vitiligo causes more distress for those with darker skin** – the idea that the more obvious that a condition is the more problems it will cause is not necessarily true. Different factors affect the extent to which patients are affected by their condition, and culture and social support have been found to be more important than skin colour.
- **Vitiligo is related to the consumption of certain foods** – a common belief is that eating two white food products at the same time (i.e. milk and eggs)

will cause or worsen vitiligo. However, there is no evidence whatsoever to support this belief; white foods have not been shown to contain any substances that will depigment the skin.

Myths about strawberry naevi and port-wine stains

- **Strawberry birthmarks are caused by mothers eating strawberries while pregnant** – as with many other visible skin diseases, food is again thought to be implicated in their cause. This is particularly true of strawberry or port-wine stains, which often have a distinctive shape and colour. In some parts of the world folklore dictates that a pregnant woman's every craving needs to be satisfied or the baby will be born with a mark signifying the unsatisfied craving. In other parts of the world the opposite is true and mothers who eat too much of a particular food are thought to be responsible for the shape and colour of their child's birthmark. There is no evidence to suggest, however, that these beliefs are true.

- **The shape of the mark has a particular significance** – this belief centres around the view that the shape of a lesion has a mysterious or religious quality. This idea may have originated in biblical teachings where having a mark, for example the number 666, suggests something evil about the bearer of the mark. There is, of course, no evidence to suggest that this is true.

Myths about malignant melanoma (skin cancer)

- **This only affects people who live in very hot climates** – this is not true. The harmful rays from the sun may be more dangerous to sun-worshippers from cool climates who then expose their skin to sun intensively over short periods, rather than those who expose themselves steadily and moderately throughout the year.

- **If I am naturally dark-skinned then I am not likely to get a melanoma and don't need protection from the sun** – although people with darker skins are less likely to become sun-damaged, this by no means makes them immune to melanoma. It is thus important that no matter what colour the skin is, reasonable precautions should be taken in the sun.

Where do many of these beliefs come from: the role of the media

One of the main ways that people can understand the problems facing those with skin diseases involves knowing how the media, such as television and magazines, can work to belittle or harm people with skin disease and how negative ideas are spread and transmitted. In this section we will cover the ways in which the media transmit messages concerning physical beauty, perfection and disfigurement, and will offer suggestions and practical advice as to how the influence of these aspects can be reduced or altered.

Children and the media

At present, our society relies very strongly on mass media (i.e. television, newspapers, magazines, advertisements, etc.) for information on a range of different topics.

It has been found that media influence is significantly correlated with self-esteem for all age-groups of children of both sexes, except adolescent boys; but, surprisingly, it was also found that there was a total absence of boys and girls reporting that the media is an influence on their body image. The authors thought that this was because the children were not aware of the subtle way that the media was influencing their beliefs about body image. They suggested that children and adolescents are vulnerable to the influence of television and magazines because they do not think about the messages being communicated to them. Unless they are taught the importance of the messages that they receive from the mass media, and how to deconstruct them, then this aspect of culture will remain largely unconscious to children and adolescents and yet still heavily influence them. In fact, some authors (Waller *et al.*, 1994) have suggested that teachers and parents should regularly encourage adolescents and children to question their acceptance of 'ideal' media images such as thin celebrities and models with perfect complexions.

The media: friend or enemy?

Since mass media began, it has had a very strong effect on society and certain standards in society; but the type of information supplied has gradually changed over the years. The media have moved from a point where they were expected to be mirrors of news and to simply report everyday events, that is reporting mainly facts and figures with little opinion. Over the years, in-depth reporting has become more and more popular, with reporters giving explanations and opinions for the events they cover. It is this change that has provoked the debate as to how much the media are actually shaping and informing society, as opposed to mirroring what is happening.

It is interesting to ask in what ways the media work to disadvantage those who feel that they are unattractive. Some people believe that the media have promoted the idea that physical beauty and perfection is a normal thing in society and that those who are unattractive are few and far between. They say that this is the reason that the demand for plastic surgery has increased over recent years, with people trying to gain this supposedly 'normal' appearance artificially.

HELPFUL TIPS! HELPFUL TIPS! HELPFUL TIPS! HELPFUL

Stop for a minute and think: 'Why are the media promoting the idea that physical beauty and perfection are normal and that we should do everything to attain this goal?'

Different sections of the media are often doing this to try to sell a product to the public and not because it represents what society is really like. Advertisers will make money by convincing people to change the way they look by buying their products. It can be very easy to be swept along with this idea, so be aware of this pressure.

Television

There has been much research into how television can portray people who look different from the 'normal' and, although only some of the research directly concerns skin disease, much of it addresses facial differences, body differences and disability. But it is important to look at the work in all these areas to understand how television operates overall with respect to those who look different: the 'big picture', if you like. Here are the results of some interesting research:

- Donaldson (1981) analysed a random 85 hours of television and noted that physically different characters were as likely to be represented as negative characters as they were as positive characters, and that in general they were not very visible. He concluded that primetime TV does not serve to promote a particularly positive attitude toward disabled people.

- Leonard (1978) investigated how physically different characters were portrayed in primetime TV and concluded that TV does firmly stigmatise people with disabilities. Of the disabled characters on TV, 40 per cent were children and none were over the age of 65. They all seemed to come from lower classes of society and were usually unemployed. If they did have jobs they were portrayed as low-class jobs. The majority of the characters were single. And almost a half of the characters were subjected to physical or verbal abuse. Many disabled characters were given 'miracle cures' at the end, and the majority of the characters had personalities that were described as dull, impotent, selfish, defensive and uncultured. It was almost as if the characters were sub-human.

● Donaldson (1981) also found that TV's depiction of the frequency of disabled people in society was also well off the mark with 0.4 per cent of characters being depicted as disabled as opposed to the actual figures of 15–20 per cent of the general population. Portrayals of disabled people were kept to minor, unimportant roles in background groups or crowds, and most of the roles were actually negatively characterised. Often the disability was shown to be the central focus of the person's life.

The contemporary average schoolchild spends 50 per cent more time watching TV than going to school, and television is particularly easy to absorb because it is convenient – the viewer can watch and listen to it. Since some authors believe that television very heavily influences young children's ideas about social reality and that they believe that what happens on TV happens in the real world, it is easy to appreciate how harmful the above negative depictions of people who are physically different could be. This is especially true of children who may not have personal experience of those who look physically different and rely heavily on the TV to 'fill in' the gaps in their knowledge.

This can lead to children growing to believe that people who look different aren't as important or valid as those who look normal. They may believe that they are not as pleasant and don't deserve the same treatment that 'normals' do. This can easily lead to prejudice and stigma and, hence, the maltreatment and isolation of those who look different. The effect that this kind of televisual portrayal can have should not be underestimated.

Adverts

It is possible that many of the images that arise from TV adverts are drawn from society at large and can be seen as a kind of barometer of cultural values and beliefs. For instance, media advertising of beauty aids may accentuate the distinction between normal and different people as they often promote the idea that attractive people have better prospects for their professional and social lives. A skin care cream may show a handsome model using the cream to get rid of their spots before they go out and have a great time, mixing successfully with members of the opposite sex, now that they have smooth, clear skin.

What this representation also suggests, without actually showing it, is what happens to the person who can't clear their skin. If the clear-skinned model has obtained so much success due to the cream then it implies that the person who has spots or blemishes does not have this social and professional success, that they are degraded and less successful than others. This is obviously often not the case.

HELPFUL TIPS! HELPFUL TIPS! HELPFUL TIPS! HELPFUL

If you fall for the message that your skin condition prevents you from achieving social and professional success you may be encouraged to 'put your life on hold' until your skin condition clears up.

It is important that you don't take this attitude as your skin condition should NOT put you off doing the things that you want to. There are many different aspects to a person and the skin is only a small part of all that makes a person. Although the skin can cause great distress, you need to remember the positive things about yourself and the things about yourself that you like. An example may be your flat stomach or your sense of humour.

Indeed, many adverts actually show this explicit difference between those with smooth skin and those with a skin condition. Of course, these cosmetic creams do not work for many people with many different conditions and so they are left with an unclear complexion and the myth that this makes them a lesser person than the clear-skinned people in society. It's this idea, promoted by many adverts, that can influence so many people and cause so much distress for people who don't feel that they conform to this beauty myth.

As the cosmetic industry expands and gradually becomes more sophisticated, TV, radio and advertising boards emphasise the need for people to control their appearance. The enormous growth in the last two decades in cosmetic surgery, diet foods and the fashion industry are all indicators in a huge financial investment in the 'appearance industry'. In the Western world, viewers are subjected to the same messages again and again: beautiful people are popular, have material goods, are successful and happy and are often loved and worshipped. Commercials can be very sophisticated in the methods they use to persuade and influence the public into wanting to buy their products. An experiment was undertaken which involved a group of high-school girls being shown 15 adverts which emphasised the importance of physical beauty; a second group were not shown any adverts. Afterwards the first group were far more likely to agree with statements like 'beauty is personally desirable for me' and 'beauty is important to be popular with men' than the second group. This little study highlights the influence that these types of commercials can actually have.

Other media

Women's magazines have always tried to emphasise faults in appearance and to highlight the importance of looking like the glossy images which adorn their covers and articles. Magazines show images of women with perfect skin and hair, perfect teeth, and perfect breasts and legs, and often serve to create a kind of stereotype which women feel they have to look like. It is often the case that any deviation from these magazine stereotypes can make many of the readers feel 'abnormal' and different.

Children of a very young age are also very susceptible. Children of a young age regularly hear stories and fairytales which pair ugliness with badness while beauty is often linked to goodness and worthiness. A look at tales such as 'Alice in Wonderland', 'Cinderella' and 'Sleeping Beauty' highlight this. At pantomimes, children are expected to boo at the ugly 'bad guy' and learn that the handsome prince gets the beautiful princess at the end. Adults have been fed these messages for years, from their early childhood through to the modern films they now see which present the same stereotypes for ugly bad guys and handsome heroes.

From the above research we can see that the media, and television in particular, actively promote levels of attractiveness and disability which are unhelpful to those with a less-than-perfect physical appearance.

Perhaps it would also be useful to investigate how the media might help the facially disadvantaged.

How can the media benefit those with a less-than-perfect appearance?

- It is, perhaps, not as important to educate the general public about the truths and the myths about skin disease passed from generation to generation as it is to tackle the characterisation of characters in the media that we discussed above.

- Recent examples with legislation against racial bias on television and radio have had far-reaching and successful benefits for that cause. Although gaining legislation for facial prejudice is less likely, it is still something that can be pushed for.

- Haefner (1976) decided to examine how powerful the media can be when influencing attitudes to disabled people. He showed that, through using colour TV announcements during prime time on three major US channels to discuss the importance of hiring disabled individuals that might otherwise be discriminated against, the intensive campaign significantly affected employers in this area. They were far more likely to hire or train people with disabilities.

- The media can be used very effectively to get messages through to the public and moving public opinion more in the direction of facially disadvantaged people. Children can be educated when young and their attitudes to disabled individuals can change. After being shown film footage that emphasised the similarities in many areas that disabled and non-disabled children have, rather than the differences, children have been reported as wanting to know the disabled children personally and as finding them more interesting.

- Television can be used to generate questions on disability; these questions can be used as part of a classroom strategy for teachers to change attitudes in children and their parents.

Television can be used to capitalise on events which provoke interest in the plight of facially disadvantaged people. The Falklands War produced several British veterans who were badly facially scarred. But these veterans, with the exception of Simon Weston, were mostly kept out of the public eye. The victory celebrations confirmed this. It is important that people who are facially disadvantaged, whether by scarring or a skin disease, are kept in the public eye so that they can provoke thought and concern as to how conditions for facially disadvantaged people might be improved. In the United States, several TV documentaries have covered the experiences that facially disadvantaged people feel. The documentaries were poignant and popular and all were well received on their initial screenings on US television.

Television is obviously not the only medium that can be used to promote the cause of people with skin disease and facial disadvantage. Dobo (1982) suggested that children's literature can help non-handicapped children overcome their fear and come to accept the disabled children around them. It was important to follow up the reading with a good, thorough discussion though. It has been shown that simulation exercises, where students had an opportunity to role-play and simulate the way the disabled person lived, brought about a big improvement in attitudes towards the disabled people from high-school students.

Hafer and Narcos (1979) pointed out that a film that was designed to inform and encourage positive attitudes to those with cerebral palsy brought about a significant improvement in attitudes toward the disabled; and this effect was shown to still be valid 6 weeks after the test. It is important to be cautious about some of the findings as other authors have found that a film presentation alone is not sufficient to change attitudes concerning disability and any film or documentary shown to children is only effective if it is reinforced by a teacher.

Culture, the media and body image

When looking at how the media influence the way a person feels about their body (their body image), it is important to recognise that there has been work which has pointed out differences in the way beauty issues tend to affect black people and white people. Wade (1997) showed how African-American males' self-evaluation was more positively associated with lighter skin colour than their female counterparts' was, and that African-American women were more successful at resisting cultural messages of physical attractiveness. This may be because women's weight is judged less negatively by African-American men than by Caucasians. A different reason could be that African-American women who identify strongly with an ethnic heritage and history that values and celebrates full-figured bodies are able to resist the media's emphasis on thinness. Although this work pertains to body image, as opposed to skin disease, it is still important to realise that the way a person feels about their body and the way they look can be different as a result of their cultural background. Although the effect of the media is important, it can affect different people in different ways.

Beauty and ideas of what is and is not beautiful are not fixed. Many people differ on what they think is attractive. The work above shows that this can vary from culture to culture and, contrary to images that might be seen in the media, it is not a person's skin that makes them attractive but a combination of all the unique characteristics that they are.

Although it deals with various physical handicaps and there is little direct work on skin disease, it is still important to mention the above research for two reasons. Firstly, The work summarised above gives an interesting and insightful set of examples to show just how important the media are in influencing attitudes to people who are physically disadvantaged and to show what can be done about this. Secondly, many people do consider that their skin disease stigmatises them and can often make them feel bad about themselves and how they look. They can feel self-conscious and often feel that people are looking at their condition and judging them negatively and discriminating against them because of how they look. This set of feelings can be very similar to that felt by those who are disabled or facially disadvantaged in another way. Skin disease is treated similarly by the popular media.

How do these beliefs make people feel: skin disease type and stigma

The extent to which a patient will feel stigmatised will often depend on the nature of the skin condition and the beliefs associated with it. Social stigma refers to the process by which a person's behaviour or appearance is considered to be deviant by others and leads to prejudicial thoughts, utterances or behaviours. Dani, a 48-year-old mother of two with vitiligo describes her experience of stigma with a group of strangers.

Reactions of strangers

❝I was at the cosmetics counter in a large department store when I noticed two teenage girls looking at me and laughing. They were being really rude and although I don't usually say anything ... I mean I don't usually react to rude remarks, I asked them what their problem was. One of them then looked at me in disgust and said, 'We don't have a problem but you do because no matter how much make-up you buy you are still going to look like a freak'. I was so shocked and distressed by what they had said that I ran out of the shop in tears.❞

Although it deals with facial disfigurement that is not skin disease, this example highlights how the anonymity that comes with being a stranger leads to people casting aside basic social norms, such as politeness and respect for others' feelings. It is common for people with visible skin conditions to be subjected to socially stigmatising reactions from strangers rather than from people with whom they are likely to have more consistent contact. The case described above may seem extreme. However, even in cases where there is no intention to hurt or be rude, the effects of stigma are no less hurtful, though the rejection may be more subtle. Anthony, a 21-year-old acne sufferer, describes his experience:

❝Me and some friends, there was about five of us, we were going to a birthday party being held at the house of one of my closest friend's cousins. I had never met this cousin before but my friend said that he had told him to bring whoever he wanted to the party. When we arrived, a pretty young woman opened the door and my friend started to introduce all of us. She greeted everybody with a warm smile and a kiss on the cheek, but when it was my turn to be introduced she just smiled politely and shook my hand. I felt that I repulsed her.❞

Chapter 4 addresses ways of coping with the effects of the stigma that can be associated with skin disease.

Summary

- The myths about skin problems can influence a person's adaptation to their condition. Beliefs about the course, cause and cure of their illness will often have a negative impact on people's adjustment.

- The myths about skin problems can be perpetuated by the media and it is these mistaken lay views that may need to be dispelled by health professionals.

- It is possible for the media to influence attitudes towards disfigured or disabled people and in many cases it is possible to use this influence positively. However, despite some positive results, attitude change is a very complicated business.

- It is easy to overestimate the influence that the media can have and, in more cases than not, some form of subtle attitude modification is more likely than complete attitude change.

- Many people's attitudes are already formed and their minds are typically made up on a lot of subjects. To effectively change attitudes, the person's thoughts and feelings both have to be addressed by a blend of rational and emotional appeals that consider the specific needs of the listener. Arguments that put the listener under pressure or threaten to isolate the listener can make any negative attitudes more robust.

- Television and other media will continue to play an important part in modifying and influencing the way many people think and feel on a vast array of topics. We must work towards securing accurate and positive portrayals of people at all points on the attractiveness scale, rather than just those who are beautiful and glamorous.

Facts about skin disease: causes and prevalence

As is case with most illnesses, the manner in which a skin disease is acquired, and the course it will run, can significantly affect the way a person adjusts to their condition. In Chapter 2 we discussed many of the mythical lay beliefs on skin disease. In this chapter we look at the facts about skin disease, focusing on the definition, causes, prevalence and treatment of well-known conditions as well as giving a general overview of some of the terminology used to describe skin disease generally.

The three broad categories of skin condition are outlined below.

Progressive

Conditions that fall under this category have a known course. Conditions such as skin cancer (melanomas) come under this heading. If left untreated, melanomas will get progressively worse and in some cases cause death. The course that progressive conditions follow can have both positive and negative aspects in terms of patient's psychological adjustment to the condition. On the one hand, because the condition will progress in a predictable fashion, patients should know what to expect and be able to prepare for it. On the other hand, however, the course that the condition will be expected to take is usually based on general estimates and may vary from patient to patient. It may therefore cause anxiety if the condition does not progress as the patient expects.

Episodic

Episodic conditions change between periods of the condition flaring up and improving. In this case the anxiety will be caused not only by the frequency of fluctuations

between worsening and stability but also by the uncertainty of not actually knowing when these fluctuations will happen. These episodes may be dependent on
specific environmental or behavioural factors, but the episodes may sometimes
appear to fluctuate at random. This will have implications for how the people cope
with their condition and the feelings of control that they have over their condition.
Most well-known skin diseases such as acne, vitiligo, psoriasis and eczema can be
episodic in nature.

Acute

Skin conditions that are acute tend to be short-lived and follow a predictable
course. These conditions require the patient to act quickly by making the necessary
practical changes to help the healing process.

Causes of skin disease

As well as differing in terms of their course, skin conditions also differ with respect
to their onset. There are two main types of skin condition onset, namely congenital
and acquired.

Congenital

Congenital conditions are those that are present at birth. Conditions that are
present at birth are usually the result of genetic inheritance and include conditions
such as port-wine stains and albinism. Some of the conditions which fall under
this category may occur in brief episodes, may be treatable and may require little
adaptation from the affected person. Other conditions, such as vascular disorders,
may remain with the patient throughout life and hence require more long-term
adaptation. In the case of most conditions which fall under this category, initially
the parents may be more affected than the infant. The way that parents cope with
their child's condition will inevitably affect how the child will cope and adapt to it
(this is discussed in more detail in Chapter 6).

Acquired

Conditions which fall under this category may be either a symptom of another
condition, as in the case of AIDS-related Kaposi's sarcoma, or a condition in and of
itself, for example skin cancer. In the former case, patients have to contend with
various issues including a reduced life expectancy, physical handicap and altered
appearance. Past reports from sufferers suggest that people with life-threatening

conditions which have a disfiguring aspect are often as concerned about their altered appearance as they are about their deteriorating health. Therefore, the assumption that the impact of the disfiguring nature of certain conditions is lessened or overshadowed by the physical significance is not necessarily true. In the latter case, the focus tends to be on the condition, its progression, appearance, spread and symptoms. The sufferer may become obsessed with the shape and size of their lesions and engage in frequent checking behaviours to see if they have changed. Since the cause of many skin conditions is unknown, the sufferer may build their own beliefs surrounding the cause and progression of their condition and may, in turn, engage in 'superstitious' behaviours to gain control over the condition. For example, someone who developed psoriasis after using a public swimming pool may avoid any form of swimming for fear that the condition will get worse.

Common skin conditions

The facts on some of the most common skin conditions, their incidence in the general population and treatments are outlined below.

Acne

- **Definition** – a chronic inflammation of the pilosebaceous glands (hair follicles that contain large oil-producing cells) of the face, upper arms and upper chest. Lesions over the follicles, which become blocked by oil, may appear as solid elevations of the skin (papules), as pus-filled blisters (pustules), as cysts or as scars. Clinical variants of the condition include:
  - acne conglobata: this is the most severe form in which large nodules and cysts rupture under the skin leaving scars;
  - acne cosmetica: a mild non-inflammatory form of the condition often triggered by cosmetics;
  - actinic acne: a rare form which occurs following exposure to sunlight;
  - acne excorie: a form seen more frequently in females, where lesions tend to appear on the surface of the skin;
  - acne vulgaris: the most usual form, where a variety of lesions may be present, ranging from blackheads and whiteheads to inflamed nodules and cysts, depending on the severity.
- **Distribution and severity** – common sites of involvement include the face, neck, shoulders, chest and back. The severity of acne depends on its extent

and the type of lesion, with cysts being the most damaging. In many cases long-term scarring can result.

- **Prevalence** – acne vulgaris is one of the most common skin conditions, occurring, usually temporarily, in more than 80 per cent of the population in some form. Acne affects males and females equally and the age of onset is usually early puberty, with persistence often into the early twenties.

- **Cause** – three general mechanisms have been put forward as causing acne:

  (i)   excessive sebum production;

  (ii) abnormal shedding of a layer of skin cells that line the follicles;

  (iii) a bacterium, often initiated by the hormonal increases of adolescence and known as *Propionibacterium acnes*, which collects in the follicles as a consequence of the increased sebum.

- **Treatment** – Treatment depends on the type and extent of the acne. Over-the-counter creams and topical treatment are usually effective for mild acne, and a combination of varying strengths of antibiotics and topical treatments are used for more severe cases.

Eczema

- **Definition** – eczema is an inflammation of the skin frequently seen in association with the allergic conditions, asthma and hay fever. It is characterised by moist red weeping skin during the acute stages and dry, scaly skin in its more chronic forms.

- **Distribution** – most commonly affects the face and the knees and elbows

- **Prevalence** – approximately 12–15 per cent of infants are affected by the so-called atopic (a hereditary tendency to react to certain allergies) forms of this condition. It usually starts within the first six months of life. Remission occurs by age 15 in up to 75 per cent of cases, although some patients may relapse later. The commonest manifestation in adult life is hand or foot dermatitis. However, a small percentage of adults have a chronic severe form of the condition, which then may be exacerbated by exposure to irritants such as dust and chemicals.

- **Cause** – there is a genetic component to the condition with around 70 per cent of patients having a family history of eczema, asthma or hay fever. The cause is thought to be related to an imbalance in the person's immune function, and is probably essentially a form of excessive or allergic response to environmental substances such as house dust or yeast present on the skin.

- **Treatment** – specific treatments for eczema include emollients, topical steroids, oral antihistamines, oral antibiotics and PUVA therapy (a combination of psoralens and exposure to UVA light). General measures in the management of the condition also include wearing loose cotton clothing, keeping nails short in order to avoid injury from scratching, and keeping the patient away from house pets and dust, which can exacerbate the condition in atopic patients.

Vitiligo

- **Definition** – vitiligo is an acquired disorder resulting in the occurrence of white non-scaly lesions. At the affected sites, the hair also usually loses its colour. The course of the condition is unpredictable, some areas perhaps remaining unaffected for years, others completely losing their pigmentation within a few weeks.

- **Distribution** – loss of pigmentation can occur anywhere on the body's surface but commonly on knees, elbows, hips, nipples, genital area, hands and feet. The condition can be distributed symmetrically where lesions take the same form on either side of the body, non-symmetrically where there is no clear pattern, focally where only a few well-defined lesions are apparent or universally where most of the pigmentation has been lost.

- **Prevalence** – vitiligo affects approximately 1 per cent of the population of all races. Males and females are affected equally and the age of onset is commonly somewhere between 10 and 30 years.

- **Cause** – no clear cause for the condition exists, although a genetically determined autoimmune (a condition where the body's immune system can attack some of the body's own cells) basis is thought to be implicated since vitiligo has a higher than normal relationship with other autoimmune-based conditions such as pernicious anaemia, thyroid disease and Addison's disease.

- **Treatment** – unfortunately, there is no reliably effective treatment for this condition. Topical steroid treatment to the small areas and courses of oral psoralen therapy in conjunction with UVA radiation exposure (PUVA) over many months are the most common therapies offered; if this fails, and failing this, patients are usually advised to use camouflage make-up to conceal the lesions. In cases where lesions cover the majority of the body, however, complete depigmentation may be considered.

Psoriasis

- **Definition** – psoriasis is a chronic inflammatory skin condition, characterised by localised, widespread well-demarcated red plaques often topped by silvery scales. In 10 per cent of cases psoriasis is associated with a degree of arthritis.

- **Distribution** – areas most commonly affected are the elbows, knees and scalp. The disease often persists throughout life, frequently displaying a tendency for improvement in the summer.

- **Prevalence** – psoriasis affects approximately 2 per cent of the population in Europe and North America but may be less common in Africa and Japan. Males and females are affected equally. Onset can occur at any age, but is most common in the second and third decades of life. It rarely occurs in children under 8 years of age. A tendency for family members to also have the condition has been noted in around 40 per cent of cases.

- **Cause** – although the exact cause of psoriasis is not fully understood, the basic abnormality is thought to be immunologically based, perhaps autoimmune, and is associated with an enlarged population of certain skin cells that divide too rapidly.

- **Treatment** – the selected treatment depends upon the degree of rash, the site of the lesions and the pattern of distribution. Thus mild forms of the condition tend to be treated with topical steroid creams in more severe cases this therapy is supported by other topical treatments such as tar-based compounds. In severe cases, topical therapy may be combined with phototherapy or PUVA, or with oral immunosuppressive therapy.

Port-wine stains (naevus flammeus)

- **Definition and distribution** – this is a congenital condition which presents as a flat, irregular, red or purple lesion. There are two types of port-wine stains:
  - medially located naevi, occurring as faint red lesions over the scalp, nape of neck or centre of face; these tend to remain flat throughout the patient's life and become less prominent over time;
  - laterally located naevi on the other hand are usually seen unilaterally over the face but may also occur on the extremities; these begin as red and flat lesions but, over time, can change to purple and become more papular, persisting throughout life and becoming more prominent.

- **Cause** – although there is no clear causal mechanism for this condition, port-wine stains are associated with a dilation or increase in skin blood vessels.

- **Treatment** – port-wine stains can be concealed with camouflage make-up; but laser treatment is increasingly available, which can often obliterate the abnormal dermal vessels over a course of treatment.

Malignant melanoma

- **Definition and distribution** – malignant melanoma is a tumour of the melanocytes or tanning cells, resulting from the malignant transformation of these epidermal cells; it is the most lethal type of skin tumour. There are four main variants of this condition: superficial spreading malignant melanoma, being the most common type accounting for 50 per cent of all cases seen in the UK. A higher proportion of females than males is affected and the condition is most commonly seen on the lower leg. Lentigo malignant melanoma accounts for 15 per cent of UK cases and arises in clearly sun-damaged skin, affecting the face and arms most commonly. Acral lentiginous malignant melanoma makes up only 10 per cent of cases in the UK, affecting the palms, soles and nail beds. It is often diagnosed too late and has poor survival. Finally, nodular malignant melanoma is seen in 25 per cent of British cases and is more common in males; in this variety, ultra-pigmented lesions grow rapidly, producing ulcers.

- **Prevalence** – The prevalence of melanoma is around 0.0001 per cent, that is, one in every 10 000. However, the incidence is rapidly rising and nearly doubles every decade. It also presents at a younger age in both sexes. This is probably because of lifestyle changes, such as the increased popularity of sunny holidays and cosmetic tanning. It occurs in all races, but mostly in fair-skinned populations and, in Britain, women are affected twice as frequently as men. Males tend to develop the condition most commonly on their backs, females most frequently on the lower leg.

- **Cause** – the exact cause of malignant melanoma is not known, but circumstantial evidence strongly suggests that intermittent, heavy exposure to sunlight is the main factor in its development. Other risk factors include having a family member with the condition, having multiple (>100) naevi, and burning easily in the sun.

- **Treatment** – the main treatment is surgical removal, a skin graft often being necessary; it is frequently fatal if treated late and a positive outcome is closely linked to early detection and treatment.

Summary

- Factors such as the way the condition was acquired, the course it will take and the physical and sensory changes that accompany it will all play a part in the way that people adapt and come to terms with their skin condition.

● Knowing the facts about skin disease enables patients to address any aspects of beliefs and self-treatment (such as stopping eating certain foods in the mistaken belief that they will affect the condition) that may have been based on lay myths.

Social coping

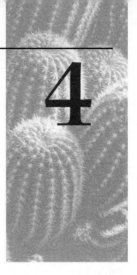

4

This chapter elaborates on factors which impact upon the adaptation and coping process. Personality traits, the severity of a condition and the length of time a person has lived with their illness are all considered with regard to the adaptation process. We also discuss the various behavioural and mood changes that may accompany the onset of a skin condition and the way people adapt and cope with these.

Stages of adjustment

Irrespective of whether a dermatological condition is acquired from birth or later on in life, there is a period of psychological adjustment that the patient must go through in order to come to terms with their appearance. In the case of a traumatic disfigurement or the onset of a skin disease in adulthood, the person goes through a period of mourning for their 'normal' appearance (Partridge, 1995). As they adjust, they may experience feelings of shock, denial, anger and sadness, before coming to terms with their 'new' face or body. The person may be preoccupied with feelings of loss associated with an image of the person they could have been (Bradbury, 1996).

There may be wide variations in how people cope with and adapt to the impact of skin disease. These variations are not simply a product of the severity of the condition, but rather they are the result of an interaction of factors including social support, social skills, optimism, perceptions of self-control and coping style (Lazarus and Folkman, 1984; Kleber and Brom, 1992). Some people may find the support of friends and family sufficient to help them cope with the challenges of skin disease, while others may require the intervention of professionals to help them cope.

Specific personality traits in people with dermatological problems have also been studied. Researchers have examined the extent to which anger played a part in the onset and maintenance of atopic dermatitis, and whether patients felt that they could cope with and manage their anger better than psoriasis patients and matched controls. The results indicated that patients with atopic dermatitis became angry more easily but were less inclined to display their anger than were matched controls. The patients in this group were also found to be more anxious and less assertive than the controls.

Coping with the disfiguring effects of skin disease

Some patients complain that health care professionals are sometimes unhelpful or dismissive. They are told, 'It's only a cosmetic disorder', or, 'it has no debilitating effects'. Unfortunately these utterances capture neither the severity nor the complexity of the sufferer's experience. More importantly, they minimise the distress and feelings of self-consciousness experienced by many patients. The disfiguring nature of certain skin conditions suggests that patients not only have to contend with the concept of themselves as 'ill', but also have to deal with an altered body image and, in some cases, disfigurement. In the field of disfigurement research, one of the most commonly asked questions of health care professionals is: What types of problems do people with an altered appearance face? Not surprisingly, given the social significance of one's appearance, many of the problems identified stem from social encounters and reactions from others. The research literature suggests that people whose appearance deviates from the norm can have difficulties meeting new people, embarking on close personal relationships and feeling positive about career goals and prospects.

It has been found that the longer someone lives with a condition, the easier it becomes to cope with it. The amount of social support a person can draw on, their social skills, their levels of optimism and their beliefs about the illness all affect the way in which people with specific stressors cope. Evidence from research suggests there is no single explanation that accounts for why some people adjust well to the challenges of disfigurement while others do not. However, the results of research also suggest that equipping people with specific coping strategies, such as those mentioned later in the chapter, can positively affect their ability to deal with their condition.

Adjusting to a change in physical appearance

In many cases, people who have become disfigured have to adapt to a new body image. They need to get used to their new appearance and learn to cope with the challenges of living with an appearance which deviates from the norm. In the case of skin disease, however, adapting to a new body image is further complicated by the fact that some skin conditions are episodic in nature. That is, the nature and severity of certain conditions fluctuates. This means that the dermatology patient may have to adapt to a changing body image. A 32-year-old female psoriasis patient describes her feelings of living with such a condition below.

Adapting to changes in appearance: a psoriasis patient's account

❝Every morning the first thing that I do when I wake up is to check my body to see if the patches have changed. I know the exact shape and size of every patch and if I notice a new one then I feel almost sick to my stomach. It's so hard because you don't know what to expect; last year I could wear short skirts, this year I can't do that any more because the patches on my legs are so ugly, who knows what I'll have to wear next year to hide them.**❞**

This patient's account conveys the feelings of anxiety, uncertainty, and helplessness that often accompany the diagnosis of a skin condition. Without the knowledge of when or how the condition will develop, the patient may be left wondering about what behaviours or actions might be contributing to its progression. Lifestyle or diet may be affected or, in some cases, particular rituals are adopted in order to gain some control over the course of their condition. Some patients who suffer from acne, for example, expose their skin to the sun for excessive amounts of time since they believe that the sun will 'dry up' their pimples.

So far we have considered how a person's adjustment to their condition may be affected by factors relating skin diseases. The remainder of the chapter focuses upon some of the adaptation tasks and behavioural changes which may result from living with a skin problem. The intention is to highlight common problems and issues which arise when living with a skin condition.

Living with uncertainty

Since many skin conditions occur intermittently or are progressive, patients need to address issues relating to loss of control and uncertainty. As is the case with many illnesses, patients may go through a period of mourning for a lost sense of normality. This may be related both to the person's appearance, if it has been altered by the condition, and also to their day-to-day activities. Lee, a 27-year-old psoriasis sufferer, describes his feelings.

Mourning for a sense of 'normality': a case of psoriasis

❝I used to love to swim, it was something that I took up about 5 years ago and was practically addicted to it ever since. At first when I noticed the psoriasis around my knees it didn't bother me, but since then I have begun to feel like people are avoiding me, like they look at me and know I'm different. I don't feel normal anymore, I feel that people are looking at me and wondering what happened or thinking, 'Oh he must be so brave to be able to swim looking like that'. Consequently, I have cut down on how often I go swimming and how often I'm seen in clothes that reveal the psoriasis. **"**

Lee describes the fact that he no longer feels that others see him in the same way that they used to before he developed psoriasis. He also indicates that he no longer sees himself in the same way and that he no longer feels *normal*. Lee's description suggests that he feels that his condition affects his self-confidence and dominates what people see when they look at him. It is important for skin disease patients not to let their skin disease dominate their lives; rather it can be useful to work on accepting their condition as something which is a controllable part of who they are. Without meaning to minimise the importance that skin diseases can have, there is so much more to skin disease patients than their skin disease and their condition is only a small part of all the different aspects of their lives.

Becoming sensitised to other peoples' reactions

One of the biggest challenges of living with a skin disease is having to cope with the reactions of others. The person may experience a variety of reactions, ranging from rude comments to questions about their condition or blatant staring. These reactions can leave the person feeling that their privacy has been invaded. They may feel ill-equipped to deal with the reactions of others and consequently may avoid or overreact to situations where this might be an issue.

What to do when people ask?

HELPFUL TIPS! HELPFUL TIPS! HELPFUL TIPS! HELPFUL

If someone asks you about your skin condition, the first thing to decide is whether you want to answer the question.

Remember that you have the right to keep your condition private, even though others may be able to see it.

If you do decide to discuss your condition, take on the role of 'educator'. You can explain the cause of your condition, how common it is and how it affects you. Doing this with confidence may provoke a more positive reaction from the enquirer.

What if people stare?

HELPFUL TIPS! HELPFUL TIPS! HELPFUL TIPS! HELPFUL

People stare for various reasons. They may be curious; they may be unsettled; or they may be being intentionally rude. It is rarely possible to tell which it is. Handle staring by making eye contact with the person and smiling. You will send the message that you are aware of the staring but that you are OK with the way you look and who you are.

The eye contact is usually enough to make the person avert their gaze. The smile tells them that you are confident, rather than annoyed, and that you are comfortable with the way you look.

Modifying appearance and behaviour to hide lesions

People with skin conditions may draw attention to themselves, not because of the skin disease itself, but rather because of the way they cope with and react to it. They may begin to avoid eye contact when in social situations, wear their hair so that it covers affected parts of their face, or choose to wear clothes that conceal the condition but may be inappropriate for the weather. Their reactions may give rise to what psychologists call a *self fulfiling prophecy*. This means that the person expects that others will react unfavourably and so seeks to hide the problem. This attempted solution may give rise to a new problem: that people notice the hiding behaviour. These expectations (of unfavourable reactions), although justified in some cases, are often the product of negative beliefs that patients hold about their condition.

Box 2. Negative beliefs commonly held by dermatology patients.

- Thinking that everybody believes that the condition has to do with a lack of hygiene or is contagious.
- Feeling that the first thing that people will notice about them will be the skin condition.
- Believing that the skin condition will prevent enjoyment of life or fulfilment of ambitions.

- Justifying to themselves that, when things go wrong, it is due to having a skin problem.

- Buying into the beauty myth that all good things come to those who are beautiful.

Structuring life around disease: 'when it gets better I will . . .'

One of the most common 'coping mechanisms' displayed by people with skin problems is a desire to treat and get rid of the condition rather than getting on with living with it. Behaviours such as taking up new sports, applying for a promotion or even getting married are postponed in the hope that the condition will be cured, enabling them to lead more enjoyable lives. Here follows a section taken from a counselling session with a 22-year-old Asian woman who had recently been diagnosed with vitiligo.

Account from initial counselling session

Patient: . . . my sister is married and has two kids . . . that is all I ever really wanted to do with my life but I have decided, and told my parents not to try and arrange any marriages until this [pointing at arms] is gone.

Counsellor: What if it takes a long time for the patches to go away, or what if the white marks stay the way they are now for ever?

Patient: I am sure that if a man was to see me now that he would not want me anyway, so I am going to wait until they go away and then I can think about letting my parents arrange a marriage.

Counsellor: It sounds like you are certain about the way that such a meeting would turn out, aren't you limiting your chances of achieving your goal, to get married and have a family, by not allowing your parents to arrange these meetings?

Patient: No because I am sure . . . . 100 per cent sure that no one would want me looking like this. When I am better, then I can start thinking about it again.

This patient expresses the view that, as a person with vitiligo, she is undesirable and that none of her dreams or ambitions can be achieved while she has vitiligo. It is important that patients challenge these thoughts that exemplify the negativity about the condition. For instance, the following questions could be useful for the woman above:

- Why am I so sure that I will be rejected by a husband for this white patch?
- Have I had this experience before? If not, then maybe it won't happen?
- Is it possible that my husband will be so fond of all the other positive things I have going for me that the white spot on my arm won't even be an issue?

Some patients attribute negative life events to the onset of their condition and hold on to the belief that anything bad that happens in their lives must be attributed to their illness. This can lead to a cycle in which negative life experiences serve to back up beliefs that the condition is 'ruining' their life and to the feeling that there is no point in trying to change this cycle until the condition improves.

Visibility and choice about whether or not to discuss the condition

Since many dermatological conditions are immediately visible to others, patients may have no choice as to whether or not they wish to disclose the fact that they have a skin condition to those around them. Other illnesses, which are less prominent, can remain private and personal matters until the patient chooses to disclose details about them. The dermatology patient may feel that this choice has been taken away from them and may resent the fact that their condition is visible to others. Adrian, a 32-year-old male with a large port-wine stain covering the left side of his face, describes his feelings about this.

Discussing the condition with other people: port-wine stain patient

❝ ... and what really annoys me is the fact that people feel as though it's all right to come up to me and ask me about it. On some days it doesn't bother me as much, but on others I feel like telling them to piss off! I mean you would never think of going up to a complete stranger and asking them if there was something wrong with their internal organs and what happened and a million other ridiculous questions. But the fact that they can see my birthmark makes them, for whatever reason, think that they have the right to invade my privacy, to put me in a difficult and awkward position just to satisfy their own petty curiosity. **❞**

It is clear from Adrian's description that his right to privacy is taken away. The insensitive reactions of others can make a person feel that they have less control in social situations and no choice about how to react.

HELPFUL TIPS! HELPFUL TIPS! HELPFUL TIPS! HELPFUL

Your experience may be that your privacy is invaded and your control in social situations is undermined by insensitive reactions to your skin condition. Take back control by having a quick response ready to counter rude questions and by making eye contact and smiling at any one who stares at you.

Summary

- Having a skin condition can impact on a person's behaviour, beliefs and, more generally, their day-to-day life. It can influence everything, from what clothes a person wears, to major life decisions involving relationships and careers.

- It is useful to acknowledge these effects of skin disease and then to develop ways of thinking and coping that can help to deal with the different social situations that will be encountered.

The impact of skin disease on relationships

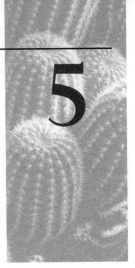

5

Previous chapters have described the emotional and psychological effects of skin disease on the individual. However, as is the case with most illnesses, skin disease has an impact on a person's relationships, which inevitably affects, and is affected by, the individual's condition. In this chapter we consider the impact that skin conditions have on different relationships and consider some of the social situations in which difficulties regarding the skin condition may arise. Furthermore, the reader will be introduced to some self-help techniques which can be learned and used in social situations.

Researchers have sought to examine the impact skin disease has on patients' relationships. One study considered the social aspects of psoriasis (Dungey and Buselmeir, 1982). Because of its visibility, the condition evokes a range of responses in those who come into contact with people with the condition. Psoriasis is sometimes considered dirty, ugly or even contagious by both non-affected people and by those suffering from the condition. This has implications for personal and intimate relationships, with patients reporting that they may avoid social contact, especially where the possibility of intimacy may arise.

In an examination of the effect of vitiligo on sexual relationships, 158 vitiligo sufferers between the ages of 16 and 79 were given a questionnaire on their beliefs regarding intimate relationships (Porter *et al.*, 1987). One-quarter of those surveyed said that they believed that their skin condition had negatively affected their sexual relationships. Between 10 and 15 per cent of those surveyed indicated that their skin condition had limited their ability to find a partner, stating that the number and frequency of sexual relationships was limited, as also were the locations where sexual relationships might occur. Contrary to what one might expect, the findings of the study suggested that the majority of patients felt more embarrassed in non-sexual interpersonal relationships than they did in intimate sexual and social relationships. A possible explanation for this may be that, since more than half of the sample interviewed were married, with an average age of 38 years, it was likely that they had been involved in long-term relationships. In these cases the issue of their disfigurement was not something new, and possibly the people who were reporting had already established coping mechanisms. The possibility of a new sexual encounter was probably less likely than a social non-sexual one. It is reasonable to assume, therefore, that they would be more anxious about non-sexual socialising. The authors of the study suggest that psychological counselling could be beneficial if it addressed problems of self-esteem and body image.

Box 3. **Skin conditions can affect relationships in several ways.**

- Family rituals and routines may need to change as a result of the illness. For example, if the patient needs to avoid the sun, summer holidays may have to be abandoned. This may result in feelings of guilt and cause resentment on the part of the partner.

- The increased reassurance needed by the patient to feel that they are still wanted by their partner may put a strain on the relationship or make the 'well' partner feel that they are insensitive and, in turn, out-of-touch with their partner's needs.

- Social contacts, friends and acquaintances may be avoided by the patient following the onset of a skin disease. This may have the effect of decreasing the patient's social support system and may place an added strain on the emotional and practical coping resources of the couple, where the patient is in a relationship.

The way a person copes with these and similar situations may depend on their self-esteem and body image as well as the social skills that they have in place.

Prejudice from professional carers

Depending on the type of skin condition, a patient may spend varying amounts of time with their GP, dermatologist or nurse. Consultations with professionals may also be problematic for patients, depending upon the reaction of the professional towards the person. Some doctors tend to make judgements about the seriousness of a medical condition in terms of whether or not it is life-threatening. Many skin conditions are consequently deemed trivial or unimportant. If this is conveyed to the patient, it may leave them feeling misunderstood or embarrassed for having taken up their doctor's time. In most cases, the first professional contact for the patient with a dermatological problem is with his or her general practitioner. Some patients feel that their GPs either do not take them seriously or do not refer them to a specialist. Many dermatology patients have reported that their problem was either trivialised by their GP and they were told to 'ignore it', or were told that there was no treatment available. This can be especially upsetting if the patient has had to build up his or her confidence to talk to their doctor. In this case it can be important to explain to the doctor just how important the condition is and how concerned she or he is about it. It is good to be able to make the health professional understand how important the condition is to the sufferer.

HELPFUL TIPS! HELPFUL TIPS! HELPFUL TIPS! HELPFUL

It is you, and not any health professional, who has to live with your skin condition. So, if you find that your condition and how you feel about it is not being taken seriously enough by your GP, ask for a referral to a different health professional.

Forming new relationships

The prospect of starting new relationships is stressful for most people. The importance that is placed on first impressions in social encounters means that this can be particularly stressful for a person who suffers from a skin disease. Involvement in a new relationship raises issues for this person about how they feel about their body and highlights their insecurities about it. Indeed, since identity is to some extent linked to body image, skin disease may leave the patient feeling that they are no longer the same person and may even lead to mood or personality changes. This may in turn affect how they react and relate to those around them. Patients bring their own beliefs and expectations to new social situations and may feel that they are expected to act in a certain way because of their appearance.

How will others see past the skin disease?

The prominence of certain skin conditions may interfere with the way that people normally behave when they encounter new social situations. The person may feel as though others with whom they come in contact will be fixated by their appearance and will therefore not be able to see past their condition. This may lead to their avoiding meeting new people or entering into new social or professional relationships. People who are unable to challenge their fears may withdraw from social activities, preferring to be alone rather than risk the possibility of rejection or social ridicule. The transcript below is an extract from a counselling session where a 19-year-old vitiligo sufferer describes how they feel about avoiding meeting new people.

Excerpt of counselling session with vitiligo patient

❝I'm quite shy so it's really never been easy for me to go out and make friends. I guess that a big part of it is the way I look. I keep wondering what people are thinking about when they look at me ... I often wonder if they feel sorry for me, if they are trying to be polite, if they are dying to ask me questions about it, but feel that they shouldn't. It is so hard to talk to someone new when you know that all the time all they can really see, or at least really focus on, is your skin! It is much easier to hang out with your family or the people you already know. At least you've been through all that stuff with them and neither of you has to feel uncomfortable .... **❞**

When do I tell them?

The location of the skin problem may mean that it is not immediately visible and so the decision as to whether and when the person will tell others can be delayed. If, for example, the condition affects the chest or the back, then these may not be visible while the person is clothed. Problems may first arise in situations where the person has to remove their clothing, i.e. when changing clothes, having sexual relations or at a public swimming pool.

It is important that the patient decides at what point they want to disclose the fact that they have a skin condition to a prospective partner or new friends. Some may choose to hide the problem by making excuses to others and some may choose to tell friends straight away; but it is always important to remember that they are in control. It is their right to discuss the condition when they feel ready, not because they may feel pressured by people staring or talking about them.

Some people use elaborate explanations as to why they are unable to engage in activities such as tanning or having sex with their partner. Sandra, a 29-year-old eczema sufferer, describes one such situation.

Transcript of Sandra's experience: an eczema patient

❝I met this really cute guy at a club over Christmas and he asked for my phone number. We went out on a few dates together and things were really going well. I was very confident and didn't even think about my eczema until he asked me to spend the weekend with him. I knew we would end up sleeping together and I knew there was no way I could hide the patches. I was convinced that if he saw the way I looked that he would never want to be with me again. So I told him I couldn't go, I made up a dumb excuse about having to babysit and work. Anyway ... needless to say that relationship didn't work out. **"**

This example illustrates how the belief that her partner would reject her because of her appearance prevented Sandra from developing a relationship. These ideas were not based on past experience, because she had avoided other similar encounters. Rather they derived from a belief that others would not be able to accept the way she looked.

HELPFUL TIPS! HELPFUL TIPS! HELPFUL TIPS! HELPFUL

If you are prevented from developing a relationship because you can't help believing that another person could never accept the way you look – challenge the negative thought pattern.

List all the things about yourself that are positive. Realise that the other person will also see all these qualities. And notice that your skin condition is only a very small part of the whole you.

The importance of disclosure may be particularly relevant in the case of HIV-associated Kaposi's sarcoma, where the condition may signal HIV infection and therefore the potential of transmission of HIV to a prospective partner. In cases such as these, the person may feel that they have no choice but to discuss their condition with others. Jonathan, a 31-year-old gay man with HIV discusses his experience.

Transcript from a counselling session with a Kaposi's sarcoma patient

"When I saw the dark purple-brown mark over my nose, I knew exactly what it was and so does every other gay man that I come in contact with. KS is like a big neon light that says, 'Hey look at me, I'm HIV positive!'. I hate the fact that I can't choose when and how I'll tell new partners or friends about my HIV status. I hate it that my skin says so much about who I am and that I am ill. Before the KS, I felt that I could sometimes forget about having

HIV. You know, just let it drift from my mind. Now all I have to do is look in the mirror or in the face of someone who has just met me and I remember …. **99**

Do others have a right to know?

Another issue that is important to consider is whether or not a person feels that they are ready to openly discuss their condition with others. Much of the research on coping with a visible disfigurement suggests that 'being open' and talking to others about one's illness may help to create a buffer against stress associated with health problems. However, some people may not feel that they want to tell others about their skin disease. They may feel embarrassed or value their privacy and their right to choose with whom to discuss their condition rather than satisfying what may be no more than the curiosity of a stranger. This experience of feeling that one's privacy is being invaded is captured in an interview with Marie, a 32-year-old psoriasis sufferer:

> **66**It was like the other day on the Underground, this woman came up to me all smiley-faced and happy, and asked me just straight like that 'What is that on your face dear? It looks painful, is it?'. I mean I was reading my paper, it was after a hard day at the office and the last thing that I wanted to do was get into an in-depth discussion about my psoriasis with a total stranger! I mean, I know that it's a good idea to try and educate people about it, but sometimes I think, well that's not my job! I mean if I had cancer or an ulcer or something internal that others couldn't see, people wouldn't expect me to answer questions about it or talk about it on the tube, would they? It's like, if they can see it then they've allowed to ask about it. All the politeness that we have when we are around someone with an illness goes out the window. It's like our curiosity to know what 'that weird-looking thing' is, outweighs the importance of sparing someone else's feelings or respecting their privacy. **99**

Marie's description of how it feels to have an illness 'displayed' to others suggests that there is no simple answer as to how to deal with the problem of disclosure. A range of factors have to be taken into account including:

- The person's confidence.
- The nature of the encounter and relationship with the other person.
- The potential risks and benefits of telling the other person.
- The predicted reaction of the other person.

- Past experiences of times when you have told other people about the condition.

Existing relationships

Although the prospect of starting a new relationship may provoke feelings of anxiety in the person, existing relationships can also be affected by the onset of a cutaneous illness. Insecurities may arise and the person may wonder whether they will be viewed in the same way as before or be as desirable as they were prior to the onset of the condition. This will inevitably have an effect on the way that we relate to others and how we interpret their reactions to us. Although it is accepted that physical appearance changes with age, changes in appearance due to skin disease are not as straightforward and acceptance may not be routine. On the one hand, existing relationships may provide a source of support for the person, buffering them against distress. However, relationships may also be a source of anxiety. The person may believe, for example, that they are no longer attractive to their partner, or that work colleagues no longer respect them.

Marissa, a 58-year-old woman with facial cancer, describes how her relationship with her husband changed following surgery where part of her nose had to be removed.

Excerpt from a counselling session with 'Marissa', a skin cancer patient

❝My husband and I have been married for 30 years. He is a good man and we've always had a good marriage. But since the cancer I've been feeling that ... that maybe he thinks I am ugly. Like the other night, I ... well I felt like kissing him. When he said he was tired, all I heard was, 'you are ugly, go away'. And it's hard to get those ideas out of my mind, I mean ... but for a bigger belly and less hair, he doesn't look very different to the day I married him, but me .... well, I am a different person. When I tell him that I feel rejected, he says that I am being silly, but I don't believe him. I know things have changed.❞

Marissa's story highlights how the 'meaning' that patients attach to events and reactions from those around them can hinder the way in which they cope and can delay adjustment to their condition. Her expectation that he would reject her because of the way she looked made her think that his remark was a rejection of her advances. Perhaps if Marissa and her husband had been able to talk more about her condition and its effects on her appearance, her conclusion about her partner's reaction might have been different. She might have realised that he really was tired and so she would not have felt so rejected. This is the reason that good communication is so important for people who find themselves with acquired conditions in relationships. It is crucial that lines of communication between partners stay open so that there is little room to assume negative reasons behind a partner's behaviour.

Summary

- Most medical conditions, whether they are acute or chronic, raise issues for the person in terms of whether, when and how to tell others.

- Some people with skin disease may not have this choice if their condition is visible to others.

- Different social relationships can be affected by skin disease. People may find themselves in a range of difficult social situations, having to contend with staring, awkward questions, and remarks from curious children. There are ways of dealing with these difficult social situations.

Children and skin disease

6

Since the psychological problems associated with a child's medical condition can have long-term implications (for instance, for the way that they develop socially), addressing these problems could be even more crucial for children than it is for adults.

There are significant barriers against children with chronic medical conditions receiving mental health treatment. These barriers can be put up by GPs and dermatologists, by the family and by mental health providers themselves. Parents can become defensive as soon as psychological factors concerning their child are mentioned and can interpret any advice by professionals as a comment on their ability as competent parents. Also, many people are very sensitive to the perceived stigma associated with health problems and family problems. With respect to the child's doctors, problems such as a failure to recognise behavioural aspects of an illness, a lack of belief in the efficiency of mental health procedures and concern about sharing their patient with another professional can all hinder the treatment process.

It can be difficult for dermatologists and GPs to properly explain the link between medical treatment and the psychological effects of a skin disease because the psychological explanations familiar to dermatologists in the past have been unacceptable to most families.

Finding less difficult ways to explain the link between psychology and skin disease may increase the acceptance of referrals and successful treatment of all the problems associated with skin disease. This chapter seeks to explore the relationship between childhood skin disease and the psychological factors associated with it and to look at the ways in which psychology can help children who are suffering with skin conditions.

The diagnosis of a progressive or episodic skin condition within the family can be stressful for both the child and the parents. Skin diseases may signal a loss of 'normality', alter the family's concept of its 'self', challenge coping methods, and lead to changes in roles, plans and dreams. Parents may blame themselves if they believe the disease to be hereditary, and siblings may themselves fear acquiring the disease. Janice is a mother of a 15-month-old baby with eczema and she describes her feelings about her baby:

> **"**When Jessica was born, I was really excited that I'd had a little girl. I wanted a girl so much that I had even bought little dresses for her before she was born! She was going to be my little doll. I think when the eczema came on it was a real shock to me. I had heard about the condition but didn't know much about it. I didn't expect that I would have to make so many changes to deal with it. You see, Jessica's skin gets very itchy so she becomes really uncomfortable and cries a lot, sometimes all through the night. I can't dress her in the clothes that I want because she has a bad reaction to certain fabrics. Also, I have to apply this special ointment to her patches, but she hates that and starts screaming when she sees me coming with the tub of cream. I feel really bad when she struggles with me like that. Sometimes I feel that we aren't close enough, you know. I can't play with her or cuddle her, because she gets really uncomfortable. It's very hard for us. It's like the eczema won't allow me to have the relationship, the closeness that I want with my daughter.**"**

This case illustrates some of the difficulties that can arise when a young child develops a skin condition. A central concern of this mother was her relationship and attachment to her child. Her story illustrates how anxiety-provoking it can be not to be able to bond easily with her child.

Skin disease and the parent–child relationship

The relationship between the child and the parent may have implications for the way in which the child makes sense of and copes with his or her condition. Research suggests that one of the most significant factors in the development of behavioural problems of children with disfiguring skin conditions is the reaction of the parents to the illness or deformity. Over-protective parents who shield their child from social problems, such as teasing, may prevent the development of childhood friendships and social skills, which are vital for later life. The birth of an infant of remarkable appearance can cause delay in how they bond with their mother and result in sadness, similar to that experienced by mothers of infants with other congenital disorders.

Normal reactions of parents, which tend to occur with the birth of a child with a skin condition, are detailed below. Parents of children with skin disease should be aware of these.

- **Parental mourning, i.e. the denial, anger and sadness that the parent feels following the birth of the child** – Being informed that one's child is ill or has some handicap is a life crisis which brings with it changes. Parents face the prospect of having to adapt to circumstances that they might not have ever imagined having to contend with.

- **Disappointment, shame or guilt** – Guilt is a common feeling that accompanies the birth of a child with an illness. This is especially relevant in cases where the illness has been genetically transmitted, but can also occur when the onset cannot be linked to genetic causes. Parents may have an unrealistic expectation of how the illness will affect the child's life. They may also feel unprepared emotionally, financially and practically to deal with the challenges of bringing up the child. This may make them feel inadequate and add to the feelings of guilt that they have about the child's illness.

- **Over-protection or over-indulgence stemming from parental anxiety** – The anxiety that parents feel about their child's condition may affect the way that they behave towards them. Parents may become over-protective of their child in order to buffer them against the social and physical consequences of their illness. Similarly they may try to over-compensate for the fact that their child has to live with a chronic skin condition by over-indulging them, causing resentment in other siblings.

- **Focusing on the needs of the sick child and disregarding or downplaying the needs of the other children in the family** – Difficulties that often face a family that has a child with a chronic skin disease are the way that the illness affects the family as a whole, and how the individual members are affected. In some cases, a parent's guilt regarding their child's illness and need to compensate for it is expressed through an over-involvement with the child. This will inevitably have implications for how the parent will deal with the other children.

- **Parental neglect or rejection of the sick child** – Another possible reaction of parents is one where the child is rejected because they do not feel that they can cope with the child's illness. This may stem from the fear that if they get too close emotionally it will be too distressing for them. It may also be due to a belief that they will be letting down their child if they are unable to help them cope. Parental rejection can also occur when the disfigurement or skin disease is believed to have resulted from sin or wrongdoing.

- **Anger or resentment about the financial and practical burdens of care-taking and medical treatment** – Like any illness, skin disease brings with it practical challenges with which the family will have to contend. Depending on the condition, parents may have to make changes to their daily routine, such as taking the child to the clinic or treatment centre. The issue of cost may also arise where parents have to find ways of financing either treatment or care-taking that the illness of their child necessitates. All these factors may contribute to making parents feel resentful of the amount of time and effort that they have to put into the management of their child's condition.

- **Parental depression and fatigue** – The factors described above can lead to depression and fatigue in parents. In cases where the child's condition is chronic or episodic, the parents may feel that they have no control over the child's illness and that their efforts to improve the child's condition are in vain. The fact that so much of their energy is centred on the child and the illness means that their own needs are likely to go unmet and that fatigue and depression can occur.

- **Marital problems between parents** – Illness resonates throughout the whole family and relationships between family members can often be adversely affected. Parents of an ill child may become so absorbed with their child's condition that they begin to neglect their own needs and those of other family members. They may find it difficult to share their feelings with others and can therefore isolate themselves from their partner and other family members.

HELPFUL TIPS! HELPFUL TIPS! HELPFUL TIPS! HELPFUL

'Negative' reactions and occasional lapses from ideal behaviour are perfectly natural and very common in parents of children with skin disease. They don't make you a 'bad parent'.

Be aware of the potential reactions you may have so that you recognise them when they arrive. And avoid falling into regular patterns of behaviour that makes the child, or the parent, unhappy.

When you, or your child, are having difficulties with 'negative' reactions or behaviour, visit your GP to arrange to talk things through with a professional.

Stress and emotions

Stress has been shown to be an important contributory factor in conditions such as eczema and psoriasis. The way in which stress affects these conditions is thought to be a complex process which involves changes in the way children perceive their pain and itching, changes in the child's immune function and changes in inflammatory responses.

Research on children with skin diseases has focused on the role of the family environment in the maintenance of the symptoms. Different kinds of stress and family organisational structures have been researched with respect to how they affect the severity of children's eczema. It has been shown that less severe eczema symptoms were associated with a more organised and independent family structure. This research is a good example of the very complex relationship between children's skin disease and the psychological factors that can affect it. The authors of this research concluded that more organised families were better at protecting their children from stress and better at carrying out treatment programmes than those that were not so well organised.

Psychological treatments that have been designed to limit the severity of skin diseases (usually eczema and psoriasis) have included different but complementary aspects such as working on the reduction of scratching behaviours and the reduction of stress. Research has shown that patients with severe eczema who received instruction in relaxation, as well as in what are called techniques to reduce scratching, showed vastly diminished eczema severity and medication use.

Interestingly, it has been shown that the use of a relaxation-type treatment has been successful with children whose eczema was considered to be resistant to the usual dermatological treatments. The children's treatment consisted of listening to tapes of 'magic music' to increase relaxation and reduce scratching at bedtime. Most children improved on scratching, itching and sleep disturbance and, importantly, a follow-up a few years later revealed that the majority of patients had maintained these gains. It is thought that providing a form of structured distraction at a common 'scratching time' for children is the route by which these treatments are effective.

Stress, and the problems relating to having the skin disease, play an important role in the maintenance of the child's condition; treatment involving stress reduction has been shown to be effective.

Children's scratching and itching: What can I do?

Children with skin conditions such as eczema and psoriasis may often scratch their skin. It is well known that scratching can significantly worsen the symptoms of skin disease, sometimes causing infection. It has been common for scratching behaviour to be viewed as a habit much like any other habit, repeated because it effectively brought relief from itching in the past.

Some authors have suggested that children's scratching may be related to social and environmental factors and showed this by asking 30 children with severe atopic dermatitis and their parents to undertake a series of tasks together which were either structured or unstructured. They found that the children were more likely to scratch their skin or ask their parents to scratch them during play rather than when they have to undertake a task together. What was extremely important about this particular research was that they found that scratching and rubbing were most likely to occur when the parents were asking the children to stop scratching or otherwise paying attention to the child's scratching behaviour. By paying attention to these behaviours, parents can reinforce scratching and actually make it worse. Accordingly, parents should be careful to consciously limit the attention they give to children's scratching behaviour. The authors showed that children's scratching and rubbing were less likely to occur when parents were attending to other, non-scratching behaviours.

HELPFUL TIPS! HELPFUL TIPS! HELPFUL TIPS! HELPFUL

Help your child to reduce scratching by:

- Paying less attention to scratching-related behaviour, including making less physical contact.

- Increasing your overall attention to appropriate behaviours that don't involve scratching.

- Encouraging your child's involvement in tasks (especially at times when scratching is most likely to occur, e.g. at bedtime, when studying).

- Minimising attempts to stop your child from scratching.

So far we have looked at some behavioural and psychological aspects of trying to improve the child's skin disease. Since childhood skin disease most commonly begins in early childhood, problems with sleep can arise due to itching and scratching. It is thought that long-term sleep problems further worsen the skin through psychological stress and it is important to emphasise the importance of good sleep for both child and parents in managing the stresses of the day.

It has been shown that children with atopic dermatitis have a greater number of night wakings than children without dermatitis. Sleep continuity is likely to be affected by itching and scratching.

Children's sleep problems: What can I do?

Many parents may assume that disrupted sleep is inevitable and that there is nothing that can be done about it; but parents must be reassured that sleep disruption is preventable and a worthwhile goal on account of all the consequences of insufficient sleep.

HELPFUL TIPS! HELPFUL TIPS! HELPFUL TIPS! HELPFUL

Develop good sleep habits in your child by:

- Refraining from engaging in elaborate strategies to try to get your child to fall asleep. These strategies don't allow your child to develop his or her own self-soothing behaviours and force your child to rely on you to establish the conditions he or she needs to fall asleep (such as excessive cuddling and time spent with your children).

- Not taking the child into your bed. This is related to more night wakings and more bedtime protests and only brings about short-term relief anyway.

- Keeping the temperature of your child's their bedroom on the low side of normal. A higher temperature is an indicator of night-time discomfort.

- Minimising other common causes of disrupted childhood sleep (e.g. night feedings).

Parents themselves need adequate time for sleep and rest at night and so should realise that they need to look after themselves as well as their child as there can be a tendency to concentrate so much on their child's problems that they don't adequately take care of themselves. Parents have to realise that when they start to undertake the above changes, there will be a temporary increase in stress as they introduce a more consistent night-time structure. But this will be seen to be worth it as a decrease in stress and an increase in normal sleep start to occur.

Compliance

Skin conditions such as eczema, psoriasis, acne and vitiligo often require treatment and medication to improve the condition. Medical compliance (how well patients follow treatment programmes) has been a topic of study in child medicine because compliance with treatment programmes is very often not achieved. Although compliance varies greatly by medical condition, compliance with long-term treatment programmes is usually inferior to that of short-term treatment regimes. Typical problems involved with the treatment of child skin disease include:

- Using topical treatments inconsistently.
- Stopping treatments when the severity of the problem diminishes.
- Failing to monitor the skin condition and hence failing to notice early signs of recurrence/restarting treatment.

Compliance with treatments typically vary with the child's developmental level. For the infant and young child, the parent/caregiver takes responsibility for the treatment. One of the problems for parents who have to administer treatment to young children is actually getting the infant to cooperate with time-consuming and uncomfortable tasks. Older children and adolescents tend to take a role in their own medical care and the success with which they maintain their treatment regime often depends upon how independent the child is.

In the question of how children adhere to treatment programmes, it is important to realise that children may be providing their parents and medical staff with false information. Another problem occurs when parents try to present themselves as more compliant than they actually are.

Several strategies exist to improve the compliance of children with medical regimes.

The administration of a treatment programme and any problems associated with this should be treated as a problem to be solved. Parents should increase both their own and their child's knowledge about the treatment and its purpose. Heffer and colleagues (1997) found that providing written instructions in addition to spoken ones during child visits improved accurate recall of the treatment regime in both parents and children. Arranging (when possible) the time of treatment application to be that which is most suitable to the patient will increase compliance.

HELPFUL TIPS! HELPFUL TIPS! HELPFUL TIPS! HELPFUL

The following strategies have been used with some success in the past for maintaining compliance with different medical treatment regimes: ▶

- Education: make sure children and parents fully understand the implications and benefits of the treatment.

- Self-monitoring: help children create a structured system that will allow them to monitor their treatment regime more effectively and regularly, perhaps by drawing up a timetable.

- Reward systems: for young children, arrange a reward system that effectively encourages them to comply with a treatment regime that they dislike.

Coping with teasing

Apart from the child's family, the school is likely to be the next most important environment affecting a child's adjustment. Children who are obviously visibly different to their peers may attract negative attention, leading to teasing and bullying. This sort of treatment may in turn affect the social and interpersonal skills that the child develops, and in some cases can even interfere with learning. Although some children are able to confide in their parents about experiences of having been teased or bullied, others may feel unable to tell anyone about how they feel. Some indications that a child may be being bullied at school include:

- Reluctance to attend school.
- Reluctance to go out and play.
- Showing signs of low mood, e.g. being less talkative, appearing troubled or sad.
- Displaying disruptive behaviour.

When it has been established that a child is being bullied, this needs to be taken seriously by both parents and teachers and immediate action should be taken by them. This may mean that parents need to meet with the child's teacher to discuss their concerns and find ways of dealing with the problem. Some schools have well-defined procedures in place to deal with bullying and teasing. It is important that parents are informed about how the school intends to deal with the problem and the effectiveness of any action taken. Children who are bullied need to be made aware that it is not their 'fault' that they are being teased. This may encourage them to discuss their problems with parents, teachers or even friends, rather then feeling isolated and attempting to cope on their own. Children should also be encouraged to recognise that they have some control over the situation and that they can rely on the support of adults in these situations. Parents can help by discussing with the child how he or she might deal with rude comments or teasing, and teach the child to assert themself in a non-aggressive way.

How do other children treat those with visible skin conditions?

Children's attitudes and behaviour towards facially different people can range from curiosity to abuse. Many children do not understand skin disease and disfigurement in the same way that adults do; they often behave inappropriately to those with the skin disease. Children are not socialised to the same extent as adults and so their treatment of children with skin disease can be much worse than adults', although much of their behaviour arises from curiosity as opposed to malice. Some research has been carried out to examine the effectiveness of various educational strategies for changing children's attitudes to people who look different from themselves. It was noted that when children were given a 5-hour plan of activities that aimed to allow them to be put in the position of disadvantaged children, significant positive changes in the children's attitudes were found.

Educating children to understand difference should be emphasised in the classroom setting as well as at home.

Helping children 'get over' their curiosity about a condition can help them to focus on other aspects of the child not necessarily related to the child's appearance.

Explaining skin disease to children

❝Samantha was a happy, outgoing 6-year-old who had been born with a large port-wine stain on the left side of her face and neck. The mark did not seem to bother Samantha. She and her mother referred to it as her 'strawberry stamp', and joked about how it was proof that she loved strawberry ice-cream. When she was around other children, they would ask her questions about it and she seemed comfortable talking about it and consequently did not appear to have difficulties engaging with other children. As the time approached when she would be starting school, her mother, Janice, began to feel concerned about how other children in the class would react to her. She decided to speak to a teacher at the school who suggested that it might be a good idea if Samantha could talk to them about her birthmark. She suggested that through this any erroneous ideas that the other children had about Samantha could be dispelled and she could take control of the situation by offering explanations that she felt comfortable and happy with. Janice discussed the teacher's suggestion with her daughter who seemed quite excited about the idea of talking to the other children about her 'strawberry stamp'. Samantha was able to talk about her mark and give a description of how it made her feel, how it didn't hurt to touch and about how much she really liked eating strawberry ice-cream and that she and her mother often joked that it showed! The other children reacted positively towards Samantha; with their curiosity satisfied at an early stage and any fears they had dispelled, Samantha was able to settle into her new class and the issue of her 'strawberry stamp' rarely came up with her friends or classmates. **"**

Summary

- The psychological implications of childhood skin disease should be discussed during the diagnosis. This often means asking the dermatologist about the different issues that may affect skin disease, such a stress, treatment compliance, etc. It is useful to list questions that the parent would like to ask before they visit the dermatologist, to ensure that they get the maximum value from their child's visit.

- Many people, even some medical staff, can have a tendency to minimise the often very distressing effects of skin disease with lines such as 'after all, it's not that bad, it's only cosmetic'. This kind of short-sighted attitude bears no resemblance to the often severe distress that can accompany childhood skin disease, both for the child and for the parent. The parent should not feel that their concern is unjustified.

- While ensuring that the distress is not minimised, it is useful for families to normalise the problems they encounter that arise from childhood skin disease. It is very common for families to be affected by problems due to skin disease such as sleeping problems, stress and non-compliance with treatment programmes. There are many others in the same situation and many people can take comfort from that.

Treatment 1: The people (health professionals, skin camouflage and support groups)

Professionals involved in the treatment of skin disease

The parents of a new-born baby with a congenital skin condition or a person who acquires a skin disease later in life may be confronted by a wide range of health professionals. In this section we list the professionals that a skin disease patient may meet at some point during their health consultation, and briefly describe the role they play.

As will be seen, the problems associated with skin conditions can be many and varied and a wide range of health professionals can be involved in the treatment process.

Dermatologists

These are physicians who specialise in dealing with skin conditions which require medical treatment. The conditions that dermatologists work with include acne, psoriasis, eczema, vitiligo, urticaria and some skin cancers. They often prescribe conventional medical treatments such as steroid creams, tablets, lotions and sessions of ultraviolet light therapy and can give good advice to patients and parents of children with skin conditions on good management of the skin. Since they tend to specialise in the physiological aspects of the skin, some dermatologists do not always appreciate the psychological aspects that can be associated with the condition – and this is where psychologists and psychiatrists can come in.

Psychologists

Psychologists are non-medical professionals who are trained to help people to deal with emotional and behavioural problems. The training they receive is based on a past knowledge of psychological theory and often includes specialised clinical training, although not always. Psychologists often work with individuals or families and, in the case of skin disease, they have been shown to have achieved considerable success with both adult and child skin disease patients. Since skin disease can often affect an individual's body image, self-esteem and quality of life, psychologists can work with skin disease patients to help them to develop new ways of coping with their condition so that the patient's body image, self-esteem and quality of life improve.

Psychiatrists

Psychiatrists are doctors, like dermatologists, but instead of specialising in skin, their speciality is in working with people who experience mental illness. For example, psychiatrists may be called upon to work with patients who have delusions of problems that don't actually exist. A common condition is that of delusions of parasitosis where the sufferer believes that their skin is infested with parasites. These patients often present to psychiatrists with scarred lesions on their arms where they have attempted to remove the 'parasites'.

Nurses

Almost everyone is aware of the role of nurses in looking after the needs of patients in hospital. Nurses are often involved with the consultation and treatment aspects of skin disease. There are other ways that nurses can be involved in the care of those with skin diseases. Nurses often have daily contact with patients and their families during hospital treatment and so may be the first professional to be aware of the distress involved with the condition. They have experience of multidisciplinary treatment, in that they are medically trained, but are also experienced in counselling skills and so can be the first to offer help to patients. Nurses have wide experience of the psychological and physical aspects of skin conditions, because they see so many people on a daily basis, and so they are often able to recognise patient's reactions to their skin disease and so can be aware of who may benefit from psychological referral.

Health visitors

These specialist health professionals work closely with the family doctor and are involved in the care of people in the community. They are often involved in the care of babies and young children, although their work can include people of any age. These nurses can be especially useful in offering advice to parents who may be experiencing feeding or sleeping problems with their children. They are also involved in monitoring the development of the children and their skin disease.

Because health visitors have regular contact with parents and the family home, they often find that they are involved in helping the parents to cope with the emotional adjustment that comes with the birth of a baby with a skin disease.

Genetic counsellors

These are doctors who have a specialist knowledge of particular congenital diseases, including skin disease. Their job is to give families information on the reasons that particular congenital conditions occurred and what the chances are of the condition appearing in the family in future generations.

Talking to your doctor

Most people have a horror story to tell about a visit to their doctor. Be it long waiting times, insensitivity or simply feeling rushed, most of us have at some point had a bad experience with our doctor. By the same token, however, most have also had wonderful experiences where health carers have gone out of their way to help us, or been a great source of support through difficult times. So why this difference in our experiences of health care practitioners? In this section we examine the complex relationship between patients and their doctors. We look firstly at why patient/practitioner interaction is important and also what factors affect it.

Patient–doctor communication

As with any sort of communication, that between patients and their doctors is a two-way street, with both parties getting it wrong sometimes. Unfortunately, however, poor communication can have serious effects on a patient's treatment. It has been linked to outcomes as problematic as non-compliance with treatment, absence from important follow-up appointments and, in extreme cases, litigation. Furthermore, although most of us are able to recognise a case of blatant incompetence, most of us are insufficiently knowledgeable about medicine to know how good the treatment we have been given really is. We tend to judge our doctors less often on the care that they give us and more often on the way that it is given. The fact that a patient's first port of a call will be their local GP when they seek help for their skin condition may raise a variety of problems. First and foremost they need to remember that their GP is often very busy and probably under a lot of pressure to get through a waiting-room full of patients – with the result that he or she may be less likely to respond to the emotional aspects of their concerns. Secondly, it is not a prerequisite for general practitioners to have any training in dermatology. This means that the GP may not actually have much experience dealing with dermatological problems. And thirdly, many health care workers see dermatology as being at the bottom of their list of medical priorities as these conditions are rarely life-threatening and tend to be seen as more of a cosmetic problem. Few of these problems are a direct consequence of the doctor's behaviour. Rather do they stem from an overburdened health care system where both providers and patients are put under pressure to meet the specific demands made of them.

When doctors get it wrong

Listening

One of the most commonly reported problems is communicating. Doctors are often rushed off their feet with busy waiting-rooms and, in fact, a famous study carried out by Beckman and Frankel in 1984 found that in only 23 per cent of cases that they observed were patients allowed to finish their explanation before the doctor interrupted.

The use of technical language

The use of jargon is another common barrier in patient–doctor communication. In some cases jargon explanations are used to dissuade the patient from asking too many questions. However, a more likely reason is that the jargon that doctors use is a carryover from their training, where they are taught a complex vocabulary and communicate this to other professionals. They can get so used to doing this that they forget that the patient doesn't share their expertise. Another explanation for why this happens is that doctors may be unclear about the amount and type of information they should share with patients.

Depersonalisation of the patient

This is another common block in communication, which may be used intentionally to keep the patient quiet and help the doctor to focus. Or it may happen unintentionally, because most doctors are trained to treat the illness and not the patient. Thus they may focus on a skin lesion and how to cure this as opposed to considering how the patient is feeling about it.

When patients get it wrong

Through their attitudes and behaviour, patients too can contribute to poor doctor–patient relations. Patients often bring a sense of anxiety into the consultation room and this can lead to the patient experiencing difficulties in attention and concentration making it difficult for the patient to process incoming information. This kind of anxiety can also make it difficult to retain what information is learned.

Another problem that the patient can bring is the fact that they often 'respond to different cues' about their conditions than do the doctors. Where patients can often be preoccupied with the pain and symptoms of their conditions, doctors tend to focus on the underlying illness, its objective severity and its treatment. Patients may not understand the doctor's focusing on factors that they consider to be incidental to the main problem and this can be the source of tension in the consultation.

A final problem that can present in the consultation is when the patient fails to give all the necessary information to the doctor, through fear of the consequences of giving that information. In the case of skin disease a good example could be an individual reporting to the doctor with a skin complaint on the arms and around the groin area. The patient may be embarrassed and fail to point out that the skin complaint is located in the groin area as well as on the arms. But this failure could result in a different diagnosis being made to the one which might have been made had the doctor known that the skin complaint was on the groin as well as the arms.

A lack of feedback can be an interactive problem between the patient and the doctor and those who do receive feedback tend to receive negative feedback rather than positive feedback. People who have left the consultation with a recommended treatment that is successful are unlikely to return; but those who feel that their treatment has been unsuccessful will return. If a patient does not return after a treatment recommendation from a doctor, it could be for a number of reasons. It could be a result of a successful cure. Or, the treatment may have failed but the disorder cleared up anyway. Or, the patient could have decided to change doctors, since the previous doctor's recommendation failed in their eyes. Or, the patient could have died. It is important to give good feedback when possible; this will only improve communication between patient and doctor.

Cosmetic camouflage

The British Red Cross Society Skin Camouflage Service, run by the British Red Cross, provides a nationwide service offering advice to individuals on the selection and application of camouflage creams. The creams can be used on all areas of the body to reduce the impact of a variety of conditions and scarring. They are useful for covering vitiligo and are particularly effective when used on the face.

Camouflage creams differ from ordinary cosmetics in that they have a greater opacity, therefore greater covering power, and they are waterproof if treated with care. The creams contain some sunscreen, but sunblock can be worn under the camouflage creams as additional protection. There are very few recorded cases of patients having an allergic reaction to camouflage creams, although some of the brands do contain lanolin.

The British Red Cross Skin Camouflage Service is available to men, women and children via a referral from their doctor or consultant. The service is provided free of charge and the recommended creams are available on prescription. At a British Red Cross skin camouflage clinic a highly trained volunteer practitioner selects the appropriate range from the five brands of cream available and colour matches to the individual's natural skin tone. Once the colour match has been found then the individual is shown the best method of application to give an effective and long-lasting result. Below are some comments on the British Red Cross Skin Camouflage Service:

> ❝It looks fantastic. I can't stop looking in the mirror! I wish someone had sent me here years ago – I feel angry about that. (Lady with vitiligo).

> . . . As we sat down he said please do something to stop people staring at me. (Red Cross adviser on meeting a man with a port-wine stain on his face).

> You get used to people staring, it's when they draw back because they see only the condition and not the person that it depresses me. Using my cover creams allows me the freedom to be me! (User, Birmingham).❞

Appearance affects our daily lives and if we have to cope with what we feel is a disfigurement, that can drain our confidence, especially when facing new people or situations.

The aim of the service is to teach individuals the simple techniques necessary to apply creams effectively, and enable them to feel more confident about their appearance.

Skin camouflage uses specially selected creams which, while being lightweight, are very effective at covering, or lessening the impact of, disfiguring marks or skin conditions on the face or body (see Box 4).

Box 4. **Conditions for which skin camouflage can be useful.**

- Rosacea.
- Scarring from burns, acne, surgery, etc.
- Birthmarks.
- Vitiligo.
- Tattoos.
- Leg veins.
- Many other dermatological conditions.

Correctly applied, these creams are waterproof and may be safely left for 2 to 3 days on the body and for 12 to 18 hours on the face. The service is provided free of charge by British Red Cross trained volunteers. The camouflage creams that they work with are available on prescription and they would be expected to last between 6 months and 2 years depending on the area to be camouflaged and the frequency of use.

The British Red Cross Skin Camouflage Service is available nationally in the Dermatology Departments of hospitals, in GP surgeries, or at the Red Cross's own branch offices. Interested parties should contact their local British Red Cross branch for further information – details can be found in the 'Where we are' section of the website on http://www.redcross.org.uk/homepage.asp.

Support groups

There are many support groups, which are organised by people with different types of disfigurements and their families. These groups fulfil several purposes, ranging from offering mutual support to campaigning for political change.

Some groups are highly structured and run by committees who organise such activities as public campaigns, fund-raising and social activities. Some groups are more geared toward offering individuals the opportunity to get in contact with other people.

These support groups tend to be directed toward people with disfiguring conditions and their families and emphasise information about the condition, ranging from updates on health research to commercial products; but perhaps their greatest function is allowing people the opportunity to meet and share their experiences. There is a list of such UK societies, along with a brief summary of their services, in the section 'Useful addresses' at the back of the book.

Treatment 2: Psychology and skin disease

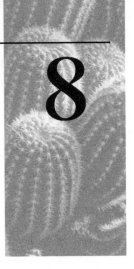

In this chapter we hope to provide an understanding of the central issues involved in counselling. We will outline our definition of what counselling is and the potential benefits of counselling to dermatology patients. We also discuss some of the most commonly used and effective techniques in counselling people with skin disease.

What is counselling?

The term counselling is often used to describe various different interactions between people, so we need to clarify what we mean when we use the term. In our definition counselling is understood as:

> **"**An interaction in a therapeutic setting, focusing primarily on a conversation about relationships, beliefs and behaviour (including feelings), through which the patient's perceived problem is elucidated and framed or reframed in a fitting or useful way, in which new solutions are generated and the problem takes on a new meaning.**"**

This definition is broad so that it takes into account the fact that helping a person in a therapeutic context does not necessarily imply finding solutions to their problems, but can provide a relationship where the person can be helped to feel understood and better about themselves and their condition.

The relationship between the counsellor and the patient is a *collaborative* one, where the patient and therapist work together to achieve solutions and explore problems. The counsellor may be the specialist in therapeutic skills, but the patient is the expert on the issues and problems that concern them. It is through collaboration between counsellor and patient (and other professionals) that positive outcomes in counselling are achieved.

How can counselling help in the treatment and management of dermatology patients?

Counselling can help patients to:

(1) Understand and accept their condition.

(2) Explore options for treatment and make decisions about treatment.

(3) Talk about relationship difficulties and find ways to cope with these.

(4) Examine psychological difficulties that result from their condition, and gain insight into what factors maintain these difficulties.

(5) Examine and challenge perceptions of poor body image and low self-esteem.

(6) Identify useful coping strategies that the patient has and enhance these.

(7) Recognise existing sources of support that may help with coping but are not being used.

(8) Learn practical techniques one can use to deal with awkward social situations, resulting from having to live with their condition.

(9) Examine issues that may be indirectly related to the skin condition but that compound the psychological effects of the condition.

Who provides counselling?

Once you have decided to seek counselling the daunting task of finding a suitable counsellor begins. We should note here that there is a difference between having counselling skills and being a counsellor. Many people who work in health care, including doctors and nurses, counsel patients in the course of their work. They do this through information-giving, clarifying treatment options and helping people to adjust to difficult circumstances. Specialist counsellors, on the other hand, are those people who have advanced counselling skills, such as psychologists, psychiatrists, psychotherapists and social workers, as well as some nurses and doctors who have had professional training in counselling. One of the best ways to find and contact a qualified therapist is by approaching the national chartering and validating bodies that most qualified therapists are affiliated with. In the UK the main bodies are:

- **The British Psychological Society (BPS)** – they hold a register of Chartered Counselling and Clinical Psychologists.
- **The United Kingdom Council for Psychotherapy (UKCP)** – they hold a register of registered psychotherapists, counsellors and family therapists.
- **The British Association of Counsellors (BAC)** – they hold a register of accredited counsellors.

All therapists affiliated with these organisations have gone through prescribed levels of training to become recognised qualified members of these bodies. As such they are more likely to be well-qualified and to practise under ethical guidelines than those who are not affiliated with professional bodies. When you contact them, ask for a list of therapists in your area who have a special interest in working with medical conditions. You can then contact therapists individually and explore the treatment options they offer.

What actually happens in counselling?

There are many myths about what actually happens in counselling sessions. We have all seen the way that 'therapists' are portrayed on television and so your expectations may be a little removed from reality. Modern approaches to counselling tend to be focused, short-term and effective. Most counsellors are concerned with helping the patient to feel safe and comfortable in the counselling session so they can explore their problems with a view towards their resolution.

Over the course of therapy your therapist will guide you through various stages of the counselling process. In most cases you will initially be introduced to the concept of counselling and any concerns you may have about being in the session will be addressed. You may then begin to discuss the problem and identify for whom else this is an issue. It is likely that over the course of treatment your therapist will find out how you have attempted to cope with your problems so far, and may offer suggestions for other ways to address the problem. Depending on the approach that your counsellor is using, he or she may monitor significant changes over the course of treatment.

Unfortunately, even though counselling has advanced significantly over the past few decades, some people are still often concerned about the stigma attached to seeing a counsellor. It is important therefore to discuss with your counsellor any worries or anxieties that you may have about being in counselling and address these early on.

Coping

'Coping' is an active process, which relies on a range of techniques used at different times. These vary from seeking social support to venting emotions and confronting risk. In a recent review by Moss and Savin (1995), the coping strategies of people with some form of disfigurement were examined. The authors found that the concept of coping was divided into the broad categories of emotion-focused coping and problem-focused coping. The former deals with the way people attend to threat. That is, trying to change the way they think about a threat and their perception of it, so as to neutralise it or make it less threatening. An example of this is where you might challenge your view of a social situation where you feel that the way you look is being scrutinised. The latter involves doing something about it, such as using practical tools for how to deal with staring and rude comments and how to confront other difficult social situations. This may include making eye contact with the other person, having a quick, rehearsed response to rude comments, or changing the subject and diverting the other person's attention. In cases where you can exert control over the threat, problem-focused coping is effective; whereas in cases where the threat is not directly controllable, emotion-focused coping is more useful. In most cases, both strategies are used both during and after a stressful event and the extent to which they prove to be useful will depend on the context in which they are used.

There are three main ways that one can cope with a stressful situation:

(1) Changing the situation out of which the stressful experience arises;
e.g. wearing clothes or make-up that hide the skin problem so as not to risk exposure and possible stigma.

(2) Challenging and altering the meaning of the stressful experience when it occurs;
e.g. if a person stares, one may acknowledge the fact that they might be staring for more reasons than their interest in the skin problem, or that they might be merely curious rather than repulsed.

(3) Controlling the effects of the stressful situation after it has occurred;
e.g. using coping skills for feelings of embarrassment or social phobia.

Counselling and dermatology

Psychological treatment for people affected by a skin disease have ranged from psychoanalysis to the use of hypnosis, and treatment methods have been reviewed for a number of skin diseases such as acne, psoriasis, eczema and virus-mediated diseases. The published literature in this field suggests that psychological interventions have proved to be effective for many different disorders. Psychological interventions, such as suggestion and hypnosis, have been shown to have the capacity to enhance immunity, and behavioural and cognitive interventions have also been used in the treatment of dermatological conditions. Behavioural interventions tend to focus on understanding and improving the ways in which people behave that might impact on their skin condition, whereas cognitive interventions tend to focus on the way people think about their skin condition. Cognitive behavioural therapy uses a mix of these ideas. One of the most effective therapeutic models in helping people cope with skin disease is this cognitive behavioural therapy style.

It has been found to help improve quality of life, body image and self-esteem of dermatology patients.

Help your therapist help you

A common problem that arises when with counselling in medical settings is that your counsellor may make assumptions about the nature of your condition and the way that it affects you, unless you are able to clearly express your feelings to him or her.

HELPFUL TIPS! HELPFUL TIPS! HELPFUL TIPS! HELPFUL

To get the best out of counselling:

- Explain what the issues are that have brought you to counselling. Try and bring up both factual information (time of diagnosis, sources of support) and also emotion-based information (I feel especially upset when . . .).

- Be aware that some people may assume that the severity of your condition will necessarily be related to the emotional problems that you are experiencing. Discuss other factors that may be affecting your mood and coping including social support and self-esteem.

- Don't feel anxious if you are having difficulty expressing your concerns – be patient and set your own pace; your counsellor will follow.

In order to know how you understand the problem, the counsellor may ask for information about certain key areas regarding your illness experience. It's often a good idea to think about this beforehand. For example, you may want to consider *what the skin condition is*, its course, duration and possible treatments that might be associated with it, Also *how the condition affects you psychologically*, coping with the condition, its effect on daily activities and on your perception of yourself? It is important to address these issues. Lack of understanding about your concerns by the counsellor can lead to problems in the therapeutic relationship and delay the benefits that you can reap from counselling.

Cognitive behavioural therapy

Cognitive behavioural therapy (CBT) was developed by Aaron Beck in the 1960s to help treat depression. Beck believed that the way people thought about their lives and the events around them would affect the way they felt. If a person had positive or rational beliefs they would feel fine; if they had negative or irrational beliefs they would feel emotionally unhappy.

The beliefs that you have about your condition can influence how you cope with it. Negative or irrational beliefs such as, 'I have done something bad to deserve this illness', or 'Everything in my life is ruined now', will inevitably make you feel low and upset. More positive beliefs on the other hand, such as, 'The illness is only a small part of me and I will cope with it', will make you feel more positive about your condition.

Negative or irrational thoughts are often the result of 'errors in processing' whereby experiences and interpretations are distorted (Beck, 1976). Such 'cognitive errors' include:

- **Selective abstraction** – attending only to negative aspects of your appearance, so that your skin becomes the defining feature of the way you look, e.g. 'It doesn't matter that people say that I have a nice body or pretty eyes, the only thing that I notice about myself is the psoriasis'.

- **Personalisation** – feeling responsible or upset about things that have nothing to do with you, e.g. 'The reason that he didn't shake my hand is because of my eczema'.

- **Arbitrary inference** – reaching conclusions based on insufficient or inadequate evidence, e.g. 'The reason that he asked me to his party is because he feels sorry for me; there is no way someone would want to be nice to me when they can see how bad my acne is'.

- **All-or-nothing thinking** – thinking in extremes, e.g. 'If I can't get to the point where I will never think about my port-wine stain again, then I'll never be happy'.

- **Generalisation** – exaggerating the effect of an unpleasant experience so that it affects every aspect of your life no matter how unrelated, e.g. 'My friend's 3-year-old daughter didn't want to touch my hand because of my vitiligo, so everybody must be disgusted by it'.

- **Catastrophising** – thinking of only the worst-case scenario and hugely exaggerating the effects of what might happen, e.g. 'If I go out without any make-up to cover up my port-wine stain, then everybody in the street will laugh and sneer at me and I won't be able to do the shopping that I have to do' (Papadopoulos and Bot, 1999).

Challenging thinking errors

After you have learned to identify negative thoughts you will need to learn to change. If you are working with a therapist you will find that he or she uses questions to help you to challenge your beliefs. She will encourage you to think through alternatives to your beliefs or responses rather than holding on to your negative thoughts.

For example, a therapist might ask a patient who is worried about other people noticing her eczema:

Counsellor: What is the worst thing that you could imagine if someone was to see the patches on your arms?

Patient: That they would stare at me and wonder what was wrong with my skin.

Counsellor: Well, let's assume that that's what would happen. Why would that be such a terrible thing?

Patient: I don't know, I guess I just hate the idea of people staring at me. It makes me feel uncomfortable, I never know what to do.

Counsellor: Perhaps if we could work on some practical coping strategies together such as making eye contact with the person that is staring, or diverting your attention to something else, do you think that would be useful?

Patient: Yes, that's my main problem you see, I never know what to do. If I had a way to deal with it, then I wouldn't get so anxious when I thought about it.

In some cases, you may be anxious about certain situations or events but you may not be sure why this is. By asking questions relating to 'worst-case scenarios' you will be challenged to examine your thoughts and apprehensions and these can then be discussed during the counselling session.

Thought monitoring

As mentioned earlier, it is not situations in and of themselves that are stressful or depressing, but rather the perception that we have of them. If we learn to firstly identify negative or erroneous thoughts and then challenge them, we can influence our interpretation of emotional reactions to various situations. Becoming more aware of your thoughts can be achieved by recording when you are feeling upset. For example:

Patient: I am really worried about going shopping for summer clothes, I'm afraid that the shop assistants will see me and laugh at the lesions on my back and arms.

Counsellor: That sounds like quite an extreme reaction you are expecting. I wonder why you're expecting this to happen. Has this ever occurred before?

Patient: Well no, but I just feel that once they take a look at me, they won't like me because of the way I look.

Counsellor: I see. Is that the way that you usually decide if you like someone or not, or whether to talk to them?

Patient: Well no, of course not. But appearance is important.

Counsellor: Sure it's important, but so are a lot of other things, including how friendly you are and how you relate to other people. Since you said that you don't make judgements about liking people based on the way that they look, is it likely that others do the same?

Patient: I guess so.

Counsellor: Also consider this, in all your past experience this extreme reaction you're expecting has never happened to you, right? Then how can you be certain that people will dislike you because of the appearance of your skin?

Patient: I see your point. Maybe I was exaggerating what I thought their response to me would be. No one has ever said, 'I hate you because of your skin'.

As you can see from this example, the sooner you are able to challenge your thoughts through questioning, the easier it is to have a less negative and more rational view of the situation.

Another method that you may use, either on your own or with the help of your counsellor, to monitor thoughts is through a structured diary called a thought monitoring sheet. The example below describes the way that a thought monitoring sheet is used.

(1) Note down the actual or anticipated event that you are anxious or distressed about and try and rate how strong your emotions are from 0 to 100 per cent.

(2) Write down your thoughts about the situation (no matter how irrational). Remember what is important here are your thoughts not your emotions. Once you have written them down rate the extent you believe each thought from 0 to 100 per cent.

(3) Make a note of what you are feeling and what you are doing as a consequence of the situation.

(4) Now come up with some alternative rational thoughts, and rate the extent to which you believe each of these from 0 to 100 per cent.

(5) Finally, reassess how much you believe your original negative thoughts; also reassess how you feel from 0 to 100 per cent.

Actual or anticipated situation	Negative automatic thoughts (how far do you believe each thought 0–100%)	Emotion/ behaviour (how bad is it (0–100%)	Alternative rational thoughts (how far do you believe each thought 0–100%)	Outcome (how far do you now believe the thoughts 0–100% How do you feel 0–100%)
I'm going to the gym and am worried about having to wear T-shirt and shorts.	I am ugly and unattractive because of my skin and others will notice my eczema and think badly of me (90%).	Anxiety, stress, sadness, despair (95%).	Most people at the gym are conscious of their own bodies, so they probably won't even notice me (90%). Even if they do notice me, it doesn't mean that they will think badly of me (85%). Eczema is a skin condition and doesn't say anything about me as a person (95%).	I feel more relaxed, slightly low mood but not despair. I now believe my original thoughts about 30%. I don't feel as bad as I did before (about 35%).

Distraction

Another technique that you can use to control anxiety due to negative thoughts is through the use of distraction. This technique is useful when you find yourself becoming anxious or distressed in a particular situation. If, for example, you begin to feel anxious while on a bus because you are worried that others can see your psoriasis lesions, then you may use distraction as a means to help divert your attention from the anxiety-provoking thought. There are several ways that this can be done.

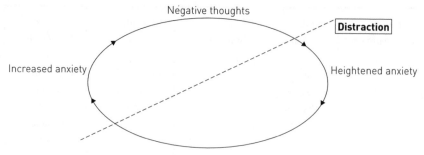

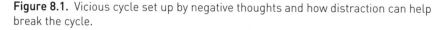

Figure 8.1. Vicious cycle set up by negative thoughts and how distraction can help break the cycle.

Firstly, you can focus your attention on a neutral event or object, for example by counting how many people on the bus are wearing blue sweaters or how many cars overtake you. Secondly, you can try mental exercises such as reciting the alphabet backwards or counting to one thousand in multiples of 13. Finally, another useful technique involves trying to recall in detail a pleasant memory or fantasy that you may have, for instance, a recent holiday. Or you could dream of what you would do if you won the lottery. Through the use of distraction, you will be able control your anxiety and in turn prevent a vicious cycle from building up, whereby negative thoughts make you anxious and this anxiety further exacerbates your negative thoughts.

Using imagery

One of the tools that many therapists use to help people prepare for and cope with anxiety-provoking situations is imagery. It is based on the principle that, if you can prepare for a situation that you predict will be stressful or anxiety-provoking, you should be able to cope with it better. This may be especially useful in the context of dermatology if there is an event or activity that you are particularly anxious about. Through imagery you can visualise the feared situation while you are in a relaxed state. The principle is that if you can feel relaxed while imagining the feared stimulus, then it is more likely that you will be relaxed when the actual situation occurs. Below are some important steps in preparing for anxiety-provoking situations:

(1) Establish what exactly the feared stimulus is and what it is about it that makes you feel anxious. For example, because of your vitiligo you might be worried about being seen in short sleeves for the first time. You may be more anxious

about friends seeing you than strangers, or vice versa. Try to establish the exact nature of your anxiety, by doing this you will be able to tailor the visualisation exercise to address the issues directly.

(2) Start relaxing, sit comfortably, and become aware of any tension that you feel in your muscles. Make sure there are no interruptions while this is happening.

(3) While in the relaxed state, begin to imagine the feared scenario with as much detail as possible regarding the location and what is happening. For example, visualise where you are, who else is there, what you're wearing, hearing, seeing, smelling, etc. While you are doing this, remember to stay relaxed and, if you feel anxious or nervous, reassure yourself that you are safe.

(4) Now try and visualise how you might react to the feared stimulus/situation. Visualise yourself reacting in an effective manner and coping well. Keep monitoring your relaxation and breathing.

(5) Finally, end the visualization by checking how you feel and contemplating what the visualisation exercise felt like.

Once you feel comfortable with this you might progress to the point where you try out the exercise for real. You will probably find that you can do this much more easily than you thought because you've anticipated your emotional and cognitive reactions to the event and have coping strategies in place to use.

Remembering positive aspects about appearance

Another technique which can be useful in coping with changes in your appearance is thinking of, and listing, positive aspects of your appearance. So much emphasis may have been placed on your skin condition that it becomes all that you see when you look in the mirror. You may ignore the fact that prior to the onset of the condition you liked certain things about the way you looked. You may find yourself focusing only on the skin disease and minimising the importance of other bodily features, or indeed the importance of your body as something more than just an aesthetic object. If this is the case, you need to try and 'look past the skin disease' and identify what parts of your appearance you are happy with. Doing this can help remind you that you are more than your skin problem and that your appearance may be attractive in other ways.

Graded exposure

The fear and apprehension that a person feels about themselves and others may dominate all aspects of their life. In the same way that a person with a phobia about snakes may avoid anything associated with the feared stimulus (e.g. zoos, television nature programmes, photographs that feature snakes), the same may apply to patients with skin disease. For example, they may cover their skin up with make-up or clothes that conceal the condition, avoid conversations about appearance or avoid activities where there is a possibility of other people noticing their condition. One way to help cope is to challenge your beliefs about the feared situation through graded exposure. This involves firstly establishing what the feared stimulus is and then constructing a hierarchy of situations that you avoid. The procedure generally involves the following:

(1) Establishing what the feared stimulus is, e.g. being seen in public without camouflage make-up on to hide vitiligo lesions.

(2) Constructing a hierarchy of less feared situations that could lead up to this, e.g.:

- Not wearing make-up when at home alone.
- Not wearing make-up in front of partner.
- Not wearing make-up when friends come to visit.
- Going out to get the morning paper without make-up.
- Going out for a drive with no make-up on.
- Going to a public place/event without make-up.

(3) Rating the degree of difficulty that you would experience in undertaking each of the items on the list from 0 to 100, where 0 indicates 'no difficulty' and 100 indicates 'the most difficult', e.g.:

- Not wearing make-up when at home alone   30
- Not wearing make-up in front of partner   50
- Not wearing make-up when friends come to visit   90
- Going out to get the morning paper without make-up   70
- Going out for a drive with no make-up on   80
- Going to a public place/event without make-up   100

(4) Once you have rated the various activities or situations in order of difficulty, put them into ascending order of least difficult to most difficult and then attempt to undertake the least difficult activity on the list first.

(5) Once you have mastered coping with the least anxiety-provoking situation and can do so comfortably, move up the list, doing the same with each situation until you reach the most difficult task at the top of the list. By doing this, you can address your negative or irrational thoughts, disproving those beliefs that led to the avoidance of these different situations. Relaxation training can be added to the exercise to help you to feel more emotionally settled and comfortable while addressing each task.

Summary

- Research has confirmed that counselling has had some measure of success in helping people with disfigurements and skin disease to cope with their problems, whether in the form of structured groups run for individuals with skin conditions, or the use of cognitive-based therapies for people with body image disturbance.

- Different therapeutic techniques, including thought monitoring, visualisation and the use of questions can be applied with benefit for skin disease patients.

- Having a good understanding of the techniques that are commonly used by therapists and counsellors can help you to make more effective use of your therapy and also allow you to practise and develop coping skills by yourself.

How do I ... ?

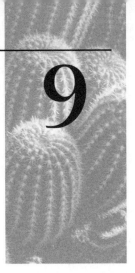

9

How do I cope with people staring?

One of the problems people often find very difficult when coping with a skin condition is the reaction of others. The first thing that we need to realise is that people stare for a variety of reasons, so we can't make the assumption that people are staring because of the condition. One way to cope is to ask yourself, 'Why else might they be staring? They might be staring because they like what I'm wearing, because I look like someone on the TV, or because they like me.' If you have come to the conclusion that they are staring because of the condition, and they are making you uncomfortable regardless of the reason why, one of the best strategies is to let them know that they are staring, but to do this in the least aggressive way possible. The first thing you do is make eye contact, and then gently smile. With this you are giving the message, 'I'm OK with my condition, so you should be as well'. In many ways, one of the most important strategies is to outstare them. Look at them, gently smile, and then look away. If you feel them looking again then do this until they stop.

   A lot of research actually involves looking at the social interactions of people with various types of facial differences. It has been found that the best way to cope is by making eye contact with people to show that things are OK.

How do I tell someone what the disease is?

That's the funny thing about skin disease. Sometimes people feel that they have the right to know what something is just because they can see it. Once again, like staring, you can make that decision. You decide whether you feel you need to address the situation. It's not your responsibility to allay people's fears or concerns.

So, the first thing I always tell my clients is that it is a private and personal disease. If you feel that you want to let someone know what it is, then that is absolutely not a problem. If not, then you can firmly but politely say that you would rather not talk about it, that you are too busy reading your magazine on the bus, or whatever else you might happen to be doing. On the other hand, if you feel that you want to enlighten this person, then have a standard explanation for what it is. Most of the time people are just plain interested so, for example, if you have vitiligo, it might be, 'Does it hurt?', 'Does it burn?', 'Is it contagious?' So you might say, simply, 'It's an illness that stops me from tanning in the sun. It's not contagious and it doesn't hurt.' Very simple and straightforward. You might actually want to practise this with someone. Have just a run-of-the-mill explanation that you give. Make it clear and concise, and, once again, if you feel uncomfortable, remember that you have to take care of your own feelings, so turn away and start taking care of those.

It can often be important to have a different way of explaining to children than to adults. Children often ask for very different reasons – such as the fact that it looks interesting. I had a client once whose daughter asked her if she had been playing with white paint, because her hands were blotchy. With children, just make it as normal as possible, and once their curiosity is satisfied, then they'll run off. The same applies to adults; many times they are asking because they have seen something on the back of their elbow or knee that resembles it. But of the utmost importance is to keep in control of your condition – this is yours, you are not a walking advertisement.

What if people are particularly rude and aggressive about my condition?

This is one of the most difficult things to deal with. Rudeness in general is difficult to deal with; but when it is directed at you owing to someone else's ignorance and is completely out of your control, it's even harder. Once again, as in other types of social interactions, it is very important to be firm with people that are like that. Remember, you are not there to take care of anyone else. Many times people are rude because they clearly have no understanding of what the condition is or why it's there.

It's also important to think about the way this problem lies with these people, because if someone is rude and laughs at you, then you have to think, would you do the same thing in the position that they are in? Then ask yourself why you wouldn't do that. That will show you where the problem lies, and you'll realise that it is not within yourself. So, it says a lot more about them than it says about you. That's always the first thing that you have to remember. If an adult feels the need to be rude, it says so much more about them, so put the problem with them. In terms of dealing with it, be very firm back, be rude back if that makes you feel better. Simply walk away and remember that it's all about them, it's nothing about you. This is so important to do because, if you start internalising things such as other people's issues, then what you're actually doing is becoming confused about what it is about your condition that is making you feel depressed.

How do I feel less self-conscious in general?

This is a tough one. It certainly can be done but it requires a restructuring of how we think about the condition in general. Unfortunately, most of us, especially in Western society, feel self-conscious when anything remotely deviates from the airbrushed 14-year-old bodies we see in popular magazines. How much more this is so when it is a skin condition that is visible to other people! But we need to remember that there is more to us than skin or than physical beauty. We have to stop seeing our body as an aesthetic object: a body is a functional object. We need to remember that there are things about ourselves that we truly value, both in terms of our appearance and in terms of what we do with our lives, our mastery of and pleasure in different activities.

Most studies done in this area have shown that various types of therapy can help us to feel self-confident. What works in these types of therapy is restructuring the way we think about things, for example, challenging the notion, 'Once my acne goes away, then all things will be OK'. Rather say, 'My acne is part of me. I'm not proud of my acne. There is more to me. But, I can go to that dance, I can get that job, and I'm not going to wait for that to happen.' It is important not to put our lives on hold and this is one way to feel less self-conscious. Secondly, engaging in more social interactions, making more eye contact, wearing the clothes we want to wear, going to the places we want to go, will make us less self-conscious. Thirdly, knowing how to deal with people's reactions, as we spoke about earlier, things like staring or asking questions, once we become confident about that, we have a tool box to take out with us every time. This gives us a sense of confidence that we can cope with the annoying little child, or the rude man on the bus. Through this, we can gain a sense of self-esteem that is reliant not on how we look but rather on how we express ourselves, how we interact with other people and, more importantly, who we are as people rather than who we are as a skin condition.

How can I be assertive with my doctor if I feel that I'm not getting the treatment that I require?

One of the things that dermatological patients complain about more than anything is that they don't feel listened to by their GPs, and, indeed, that they don't receive the right referrals. Not surprisingly, this is not the case just with dermatological patients but with a lot of people attending general practices. Doctors are busy and long waiting lists mean that the quicker the type of treatment, the better. Because skin diseases aren't life-threatening and aren't seen as something that should significantly cause quality of life problems, when in fact they often do, doctors will dismiss them and say, 'There's nothing that can be done about it. Go home and go on living your life.' What the patient needs to do in this case is be very clear with the doctor about what they want. For example, one of the things it would be very useful to do is make a list of everything you want to ask your doctor. So when you go in for your appointment you won't feel flustered or nervous, which would could cause you to forget things. If the doctor hasn't answered your questions, gently and assertively say to him or her that they need to clarify a few points for you. If your doctor refuses to give you a referral, it is important to put across your side of the situation. Explain, for example, that you understand that it is not life-threatening, that eczema won't hurt you or kill you, but that it is affecting your quality of life, that it is affecting your ability, for example, to go swimming the way that you used to, wear the clothes that you like to. Help him or her see your side of the story. Be insistent about getting a referral. In most cases, this will work. In cases where it doesn't work and your GP says, 'No', what you can do is contact dermatology societies directly, for example the societies for vitiligo and psoriasis. But nine times out of ten, if you are able to put your point across to your doctor, if you explain to him or her how you are feeling, not how you are supposed to be feeling, or how other people feel, and ask the right questions, you should get a referral.

How do I cope with my partner if I don't feel attractive any more?

Sometimes conditions aren't immediately visible. So when we meet that cute guy at the club and he says, 'Let's go out at night', or whatever, we think, 'Oh, gosh. Now he's going to see the lesion on my thigh, or my bust, or whatever the case may be.' So how do I tell? When do I tell? And, even if I'm married, how can I be sure that when my wife touches me she's doing it because she wants to and not out of a sense of duty? In both cases it's about communication. Be very aware that we don't do something called mind-reading. This is one of the things that frequently happens with a lot of depressive conditions as well as dermatological conditions. We make assumptions about what people think. We assume that the cute guy will run away screaming as soon as he sees the vitiligo patch on our leg. We assume that our wife, who has been happily married to us for the last 10 years, all of a sudden can't see beyond the psoriasis patch on our knee and is holding her breath while kissing us. Don't make assumptions. Clarify.

The first thing you need to decide is what to tell someone, like anything in a relationship. There are lots of things that we decide to tell people at different stages when meeting them. So, when do I tell this new guy that I was married before? When do I tell this new guy that I'm allergic to peanuts? When do I tell this new guy that I have vitiligo? So you need to make that decision the same as you make any other one. That'll obviously depend on where you think the relationship is going, why you think this other person should know, and how it'll make you feel for them to know. Once you've made a decision to tell them, giving facts as matter-of-factly as possible is often the best way. So, for example, what you might do is explain: that these are conditions that I developed as a child; it doesn't hurt; it's not contagious; it prevents me from tanning; and I have it on my leg. That's it. And do you think that the guy isn't conscious about the hairy back, or the hairy bum? And imagine how you'd feel if someone came up to you and said, 'I've got this thing where I don't tan in the sun, I've got a patch on my leg'. How would you feel about that? Would you suddenly think, 'Oh, you're not attractive, I don't like you'? If that's something that you can live very comfortably with then assume that your partner can too.

If it's OK with you, then it's usually OK with them. And if it's not, then this is a good thing that you know that, rather than stalling with them. But, most importantly, do not mind-read, don't stop the relationship or avoid it, just because you think that the person is going to react in a certain way.

The other thing that you might want to do is let them touch it. It may not be very comfortable, like people touching your cellulite; it's still a part of you. And once you feel comfortable with it, you'll enjoy active lovemaking or holding hands or kissing, and not let this disease get in the way.

Now, if you are married, we know that illness can affect the family as a whole. So, many times when people come to me with these worries, one of the first things that comes to my mind is, 'I wonder if your partner is afraid to touch you because they don't know how you'll feel'. Many times both partners want the exact same thing, they want things to be the way they were, they want to be able to just have fun, fight and frolic. But, because both of them are afraid to talk about it, one might assume that they don't want to be touched, the other is assuming that the other person doesn't want to touch them. It actually leads to a lot of confusion. So, once again, be very clear about your anxieties. Say, 'I'm afraid now that I've got this psoriasis that you don't find me very attractive'. And the other person might come back with, 'I'm afraid to touch you because I don't think you feel comfortable with being touched'. And in many cases it's a great opportunity to really explore each other, to explore your bodies and what you enjoy about each other, to explore what it is that you love about each other. And assume that you've married someone for more than their skin, and they've married you for more than your skin. It's important to communicate that to each other.

Where can I get advice on camouflage make-up?

The Red Cross is usually your best bet. Various different societies will offer classes and information. At the back of the book there's a list of different dermatological societies. The best thing to do is get expert advice on this, however, because there are thousands of different colours and people can actually mix them perfectly. There are also different ways to apply the make-up. So, in most cases, what will be offered is a one-off course where you sit down with a professional, your skin colour is matched, both for summer and for winter, and they'll show you how to apply the camouflage with the right powders and make-ups. See Chapter 7 for more information.

Where can I find someone with the same condition to talk to?

Once again, your best bet is to approach the various societies that exist. You might use the contact details given at the back of this book, or you might even find an international audience now over the Internet. You must be careful on the Internet, however, about sites that aren't official and about people supplying information – remember this is not confirmed information. Also, sometimes, your GP or dermatologist is aware of special interest groups that may be held at your local hospital or GP surgery that you might be interested in. So go out there, do your fact-finding, and that usually does it. Again, see Chapter 7.

How do I find a therapist or counsellor to talk to?

This is a hard one – most of us don't know what therapy actually is, let alone how to go about finding it, or knowing what a good therapist is. A good rule of thumb is to make sure that the practice is regulated by a governing body. In the UK there are the British Psychological Society, the British Association of Counsellors and the United Kingdom Chartered Psychotherapists. They will have a list of psychology services in your area. They should also let you know where their interests lie. For example, there are some psychologists out there who deal specifically with medical conditions, and some who deal with dermatological conditions; you should be able to get hold of these people. Now, this is if you want to get hold of private therapy. In many cases you can get there on the NHS by approaching your GP and explaining to them that you would like to see someone for counselling. The upside of this is that it's free; the downside is that you usually have to wait for 10–13 weeks. But in many cases the treatment is very good, and free, which can't be bad.

How do I know which herbal cures are actually useful?

There has been a lot of controversy in recent years over herbal cures and medical conditions as a whole. The main reason for this is because there are a lot of charlatans out there, people who promise miracle cures but don't deliver anything of substance. It's therefore very important in the case of doctors or psychologists that you know these people are registered. There are societies that exist that can tell you whether these people are registered practitioners of medicine and pharmacology. You should always check which your GP before taking any herbal medicines. This is imperative. These can often interfere with other medications you are taking and, instead of having a positive effect, will actually have a negative effect on you. Be aware of what you read in the back of magazines. If there was a genuine cure for these conditions be assured too that, your consultant or GP would be aware of it. Be assured too that, if the right tests and trials had been done, they would know about it.

What's the best type of psychological treatment that I could have?

At present, it seems to be cognitive behaviour therapy that is helping people cope with the condition. However, there are currently trials running which are looking at different types of therapy, both in group and individual format. Ultimately, a good rule of thumb is that the best type of therapy for you is the type of therapy that makes you feel best. That's difficult to know before you go into it. One piece of advice that we can give is that cognitive behaviour therapy has very good results in helping people cope with several conditions. It is something that is practised by most psychologists working within the NHS. Following on from that, however, it is likely that humanistic therapies and other types of psychotherapies are also inclined to be useful. But you need to look at them. We can't comment on these for sure until the results are in.

Likewise, different types of hypnotherapy have been found extremely useful in pruritic conditions. Hypnotherapists should also be checked out to find if they are registered.

How do I explain my child's condition to them?

Depending on the child's age, they will have a different ability to understand abstract concepts. Up to age 11, children are very concrete. So, even abstract things like 'forever' and 'never' are very difficult to grasp. 'I've been waiting for this Barbie doll forever,' seems like a reasonable thing if Christmas is far away. So knowing that they're going to live with a condition forever doesn't necessarily mean that they understand what that means. When we explain to kids, we need to explain in language that is as simple and clear as possible. We also need to check out with them what they've understood. So, one of the techniques that we often use is that we give an explanation and we ask them to explain it back to us. So, if the child has a port-wine stain and they come and say, 'Mummy, what is this red thing on my face?', we can explain it in terms of it being a special strawberry mark which was given to them when they were born and they get to keep it for ever and ever and ever, meaning the next day and the next day and the next day. And then we ask them to explain it back. If the child says, 'I want it to go away, I hate it,' that's an opportunity to look at doing some type of pre-therapy with kids. Why do they want it to go away? Why is it a problem? Many times it's a problem because, you know, Suzie and Amy don't have it and I do. And that's a very important time to put a positive note, as much as possible, on the condition. So, they can define someone as being special rather than being different – to know that Suzie and Amy have things that make them special as well. We all have things that we think about like that. We also need to be as positive as possible. What does it stop you from doing? You can still swim and play with Barbie and play with your friends and that's fantastic, it's not stopping you from doing anything, as a matter of fact it's a really special thing.

Rule of thumb number one is make sure you're talking in the right perspective for the developmental stage of the child. Number two is don't make assumptions about your child having a problem with this. Number three is to make sure the child explains back to you what they have understood and leave room for open dialogue. Whatever they feel like talking about, make sure that you are there to allay concerns. Number four, get rid of any myths: we know that myths abound and kids are very prone to these.

How do I become more patient and understanding with my child?

This is a question that is asked by parents whether or not they have children with skin disease. There is always a time, no matter how much we love our kids, when they're crying or nagging or whatever else it is, and we just feel that we can't cope. And one of the best ways to cope with this is to remember that it's OK to feel like screaming once in a while. It's absolutely perfectly normal. It doesn't make you a bad parent; it doesn't make you a bad person.

How can I help my child to cope?

It's one of the hardest things. Parents often say, 'I wish it was me and not my child,' and that's understandable. We hope that everything in their life goes perfectly and wonderfully, so when they come home from school for the first time crying, because little Johnny pulled their pigtails or whatever, it's distressing. As in the case of adults, helping them cope is a lot about giving them a toolbox of social skills and self-esteem skills that can help them. So, as discussed earlier, things like staring and asking questions can be overcome by a child explaining to peers what their condition is. Schools who have a child who has a severe handicap or disfigurement will often bring the child to the head of the class and let them explain what happened to their finger, their arm, their eye, whatever the case may be. This gives other children the opportunity to ask questions, it demystifies the whole experience, and it lets people see at first-hand what the condition is.

Sometimes it's not just about social skills, sometimes it's about itchiness, and we know a lot of conditions are hard to deal with like that. As adults, we understand that we shouldn't scratch because the condition gets worse; but children's need for immediate gratification is outweighed by this. There are lots of behavioural techniques that you can use, for example finding games that children can play with their hands, rewarding them for not scratching, helping them put on lotion in a fun way so they get to draw their name on their arm with their finger while they're putting on the lotion, getting fun gloves and mitts to wear at night so that when they're sleeping they don't subconsciously scratch. These are covered in detail in Chapter 6.

The other thing that's so important to remember is that we shouldn't transfer our concerns onto our children. I often see parents whose children are fine, but whose own anxieties are rampant. It is very important that you are aware of this. Children are very resilient, they're very good at coping. Although you should always help kids, you shouldn't pathologise the condition too much because this pathologises their ability to cope with it. Be able to separate your issues from theirs; be able to ask yourself, 'Why am I anxious about this? Has my child actually ever said, "I'm worried about going swimming"? Why am I assuming that there is a problem?' So be clear about where the problem lies and, if you are the one who has the issue then, again, you can speak about it with your psychologist or your GP.

I feel that I've been discriminated against in the workplace. What can I do about that?

The Anti-Discrimination Act 1999 makes it an offence to discriminate against people on the grounds of facial or any other sort of visible disfigurement. So, make sure you know your rights – that's the first thing. Be clear about why discrimination is happening. Know who to call on in terms of human resources. And, dealing with the emotional aspect of it, it's about them and not about you. Ask yourself if it's a job you want to be working in. If it is, then there are steps you can take. Remember, discrimination is not allowed.

What should I do if I want therapy but my culture doesn't approve of it, my family doesn't approve of it?

If you're living in an Asian family, for instance, and you are outcast because you have this vitiligo, for whatever reasons you think you have it, it's a stigmatisation. The last thing you want to do is outcast yourself even further by taking a medical or psychological approach which again the family don't approve of.

Having said that, however, there are times when we can't cope on our own. And many dermatological societies have special interest groups for different races now. For example, The Vitiligo Society has Asian support, and many other societies are following this lead. It's important to remember that we may feel that we should always be true to our group's culture systems, but many times these may not be useful today as they would have been in another era, another time and place. It is important to remember that, just because we go against the culture, it doesn't mean that we don't respect it. Perhaps it says that we respect ourselves and that we put ourselves first sometimes.

The family may find it difficult to understand in the beginning, but as time goes on, if they notice a real improvement in yourself and the way you feel about yourself, then they may come round in the same way you have. Their main concern is probably still how you feel.

And don't forget, if you choose not to tell them, then that's OK. Counselling is completely confidential. A lot of people come to counselling feeling guilty or uncomfortable about it.

What if I see now and again adverts to go to research? What does research mean? Would I be a guinea pig?

A lot of people who have conditions and who are with charities and societies will often see advertisements and newsletters to ask them to take part in research. Research is an integral part of any treatment process to find out what works and what doesn't work. Having said that, the whole notion of this book is about putting yourself first and feeling in charge. Don't feel that you are letting anyone down by not doing this; don't feel compelled to if you don't want to. Likewise, if you do want to, don't feel compelled not to.

Another good strategy when you see some sort of research and you are considering possibly doing it, but you're not sure whether you really want to, is to realise that you don't have to go in there and make a commitment straight away. You can just phone them up and ask them to send you some more information, so you can look at it in your own time without feeling pressured or hassled into doing something you don't want to. Just get more information through the post.

Useful addresses

The Acne Support Group, PO Box 230, Hayes, Middlesex, UB4 0UT. The ASG provides up-to-date information about acne and rosacea and has a newsletter. It was founded by Dr Tony Chu, a dermatologist, in 1993 and has over 6000 members.

BACUP, 3 Bath Place, Rivington Street, London, EC2A 3JA. Tel: Info: 0800 181199 or 020 7613 2121. Counselling: 020 7696 9000. Provides professional information over the phone and also creates leaflets on different aspects of cancer. Founded in the early 1980s it also houses a counselling service.

Cancerlink, 17 Britannia Place, London, WC1X 9JN, UK. Tel: 020 7833 2451. Provides information on cancer and opportunities for groups and individuals to network. It also runs courses and workshops on different aspects of cancer care and self-help.

Changing Faces, 1 & 2 Junction Mews, Paddington, London, W2 1PN. Provides advice and information, counselling and social skills on a wide range of disfiguring conditions, whatever the cause. Founded by burns survivor, James Partridge, in 1992.

Disfigurement Guidance Centre, PO Box 7, Cupar, Fife, KY15 4PF. Tel: 0133 331 2350. Founded in the 1960s, the centre is administered by Doreen and Peter Trust. They provide information and advice, especially concerning birthmarks, and raise money via the charity Laserfair for laser therapy.

Let's Face It, 14 Fallowfield, Yately, Hampshire, GU26 6LV. Provides a support network around the UK and in other countries for people with facial disfigurements, especially after cancer treatment. They have a regular newsletter and were founded by Christine Piff after her experience of facial cancer.

Lupus UK, St James House, Eastern Road, Romford, Essex, RM1 3NH, Tel: 01708 731251. A self-help group, run by volunteers of whom the majority have Lupus, who hope to use their own experiences of the illness to assist those newly diagnosed in understanding their condition, and to provide support to those with established disease.

Naevus, 58 Necton Road, Wheathampstead, St Albans, Herts, UK. Tel: 01582 832853. Provides information on all forms of birthmark. A support network of parents meets biannually.

National Eczema Society, Hill House, Highgate Hill, London N19 5NA. Tel: 020 7281 3553. Provides telephone advice and information; support through a national network of regional telephone contacts and groups throughout the UK; and a joint holiday programme with the National Asthma Campaign, with provision for children, teenagers and young adults. Also has a network of local volunteer contact persons.

The Psoriasis Association, Milton House, 7 Milton Street, Northampton, NN2 7JG. Tel: 01604 711129. Provides a range of information leaflets, newsletters, help and advice. Has regional groups around the country.

The Psoriatic Arthropathy Alliance, PO Box 111, St Albans, Herts, AL2 3JO. Tel: 0870 7703212. Main activity is an Education and Information Programme which includes *Skin 'n' Bones Connection* journal, Psoriatic Care Fact File and various information leaflets/booklets. Also produces a journal (two issues per year), information sheets, conference(s), educational information days and patient focus groups.

The Vitiligo Society, 125 Kennington Road, London, SE11 6SF. Tel: 0800 018 2631. Provides support and advice, produces a regular newsletter, *Dispatches* and holds meetings to which professionals from a range of health services are provided. Also sponsors medical research.

The All-Party Parliamentary Group on Skin, 3/19 Holmbush Road, London, SW15 3LE. A formally constituted group of MPs, peers and non-parliamentarians interested in skin health, which meets in the House of Commons six times per year. The APGS has held four enquiries into dermatological health care in the UK and is currently taking evidence for an enquiry into primary care dermatology services.

References and suggested further reading

Barden, R.C. (1990). Clinical management of the cleft lip/palate patient. In M. Green and R. J. Haggarty (eds), *Ambulatory Pediatrics* (5th edn). New York: Harcourt Brace Jovanovich.

Beck, A. (1976). *Cognitive Therapy and Emotional Disorders*. New York: New American Library.

Beckman, H., and Frankel, R. (1984). The effect of physician behaviour on the collection of data. *Annals of Internal Medicine*, **101**, 692–696.

Bradbury, E. (1996). *Counselling People with Disfigurement*. London: BPS Books.

Dobo, P.J. (1982). Using literature to change attitudes toward the handicapped. *Reading-Teacher*, **36**(3), 290–292.

Donaldson, J. (1981). The visibility and image of handicapped people on television. *Exceptional Children*, **47**, 413–416.

Dungey, R.K., and Buselmeir, T.J. (1982). Medical and psychosocial aspects of psoriasis. *Health and Social Work*, 140–147.

Gawkrodger, D.J. (1997). Transplantation of melanocytes. Unpublished research, University of Sheffield.

Ginsburg, I.H., Prystowsky, J.H., Kornfeld, D.S., and Wolland, H. (1993). Role of emotional factors in adults with atopic dermatitis. *International Journal of Dermatology*, **32**, 656–660.

Greismer, R.D. (1978). Emotionally triggered disease in dermatological practice. *Psychiatric Annals*, **8**, 49–56.

Haefner, J. (1976). Can TV advertising influence employers to hire or train disadvantaged persons? *Journalism Quarterly*, **53** (2), 95–102.

Hafer, M., and Narcos, M. (1979). Information and attitudes towards disability. *Rehabilitation Counselling Bulletin*, **23**(2), 95–102.

Kleber, R.J., and Brom, D. (1992). *Coping with Trauma: Theory, Prevention and Treatment*. Amsterdam: Swets & Zeitlinger.

Lazarus, R.S., and Folkman, S. (1984). *Stress Appraisal and Coping*. New York: Springer.

Leonard, B. (1978). Impaired view, Television portrayal of handicapped people. Unpublished Doctoral Dissertation, Boston University.

Marks Greenfield. P. (1984). *Mind and Media: The Effects of Television, Video Games and Computers*. Cambridge, MA: Harvard University Press.

Moss, C., and Savin, J. (1995). *Dermatology and the New Genetics*. London: Blackwell Science.

Papadopoulos, L., and Bor, R. (1999). *Psychological Approaches to Dermatology*. London: BPS Books.

Polce-Lynch, M., Myers, B., Kliewer, W., and Kilmartin, C. (2001). Adolescent self-esteem and gender: Exploring relations to sexual harassment, body image, media influence, and emotional expression. *Journal of Youth and Adolescence*, **30**, 225–244.

Partridge, J. (1995). *Changing Faces: The Challenge of Facial Disfigurement*. London: Penguin.

Porter, J.R., Beuf, A., Lerner, A., and Nordlund, J. (1986). Psychosocial effects of vitiligo: a comparison of vitiligo patients with 'normal' controls, with psoriasis patients and with patients with other pigment disorders. *Journal of the American Academy of Dermatology*. **15**, 220–224.

Porter, J.R., Beuf., A., Lerner, A., and Nordlund, J. (1987). Response to cosmetic disfigurement: Patients with vitiligo. *Cutis*, **39**, 493–494.

Wade, P. (1997). *Race and Ethnicity in Latin America*. Chicago: Pluto Press.

Waller, G., Shaw, J., Hamilton, K., and Baldwin, G. (1994). Beauty is the eye of the beholder: Media influence on the psychopathology of eating problems. *Appetite*, **23**(3), 287.

Index

John Wiley & Sons
publish a wide range of groundbreaking **books, journals** and **online resources**
in many areas...

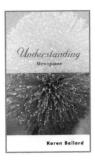
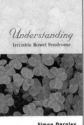
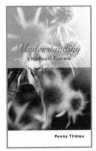
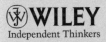